Pharma-Standard Supplements

Clinical Use

Pharma-Standard Supplements

Clinical Use

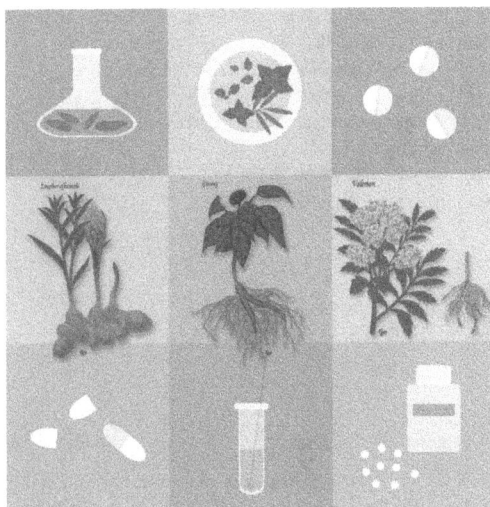

Gianni Belcaro
IRVINE³ LABS, Chieti University, Italy

Imperial College Press

Published by

Imperial College Press
57 Shelton Street
Covent Garden
London WC2H 9HE

Distributed by

World Scientific Publishing Co. Pte. Ltd.
5 Toh Tuck Link, Singapore 596224
USA office: 27 Warren Street, Suite 401-402, Hackensack, NJ 07601
UK office: 57 Shelton Street, Covent Garden, London WC2H 9HE

Library of Congress Cataloging-in-Publication Data
Names: Belcaro, G. (Gianni), author.
Title: Pharma-standard supplements : clinical use / Gianni Belcaro.
Description: New Jersey : Imperial College Press, 2016.
Identifiers: LCCN 2015049359| ISBN 9781783269334 (hc : alk. paper) |
     ISBN 9781783269341 (pbk : alk. paper)
Subjects: | MESH: Plant Extracts--therapeutic use | Dietary Supplements |
     Plant Extracts--pharmacology
Classification: LCC RS160 | NLM QV 766 | DDC 615.3/21--dc23
LC record available at http://lccn.loc.gov/2015049359

British Library Cataloguing-in-Publication Data
A catalogue record for this book is available from the British Library.

Desk Editors: Anthony Alexander/Mary Simpson

Typeset by Stallion Press
Email: enquiries@stallionpress.com

This book is dedicated to:
Dr R. S. Porter and Dr J. L. Kaplan,
Editors of the *Merck Manual of Diagnosis and Therapy*
(Merck Sharp & Dohme Corp.).
The best book in medicine.

Preface

Plant-based medicine has never been static and oriented to the past. On the contrary, it has always benefited from technological advances. Thus, the discovery of distillation replaced fumigations with essential oils and complemented water-based preparations like teas and decoctions with alcohol preparations like elixirs.

In a similar way, the spectacular advances in the realm of phytochemistry and molecular biology have nowadays substantially replaced medicinal plants and the simple kitchen-style preparations thereof (decoctions, teas) with standardized extracts and drug-inspired formulations. Ideally, an extract should preserve and magnify the activity of a plant in terms of potency, at the same time minimizing its side effects (miracle cures devoid of side effects are an abstraction). To this purpose, standardization, i.e., knowledge on the nature and the concentration of specific compounds, is of critical relevance.

Botanical extracts act because they contain specific compounds that modulate certain metabolic or physiological networks in a specific way, generally acting on several end points and in combination. Reducing the activity of botanical extracts to a single constituent is derogatory for plant-based medicine. If activity can indeed be related to a specific constituent, it will be more reasonable to use it as a pure compound, as it has been done for the so-called heroic drugs, i.e., a plant whose activity for a specific condition is essentially due to a specific constituent. Opium has nowadays been replaced by morphine, belladonna by atropine and foxglove by its purified saponins.

On the other hand, the activity of most medicinal plants cannot be traced back to a single constituent and mechanism of action, rather resulting from the combined action of a bouquet of constituents and a bouquet of mechanisms. Just like vanilla smells much better than vanillin, so extracts are often better than their single constituents in terms of potency, tolerability or both. Hemp-based medicine is a striking example. Pure THC as an anti-emetic agent has a low compliance in patients because of its psychotropic and anxiogenic activity. Patients prefer marijuana because another cannabinoid, CBD, moderates the side effects of THC and complements its activity.

In plant medicine, the mathematic relationships are skewed, and $-2 + 2$ does not generally mean 4. So, gingko is not ginkgolides or flavonoids, but a combination of the two, curcumin is not molecular curcumin, but a combination of three curcuminoids, boswellia is not a single triterpenoid acid like AKBA, but a combination of dozens of them.

This book is an attempt to address these issues under a rigorous medicinal perspective. There is no shortage of books on medicinal plants written by phytochemists, but there is a shortage of books written by clinicians with hands-on experience in the use of plant extracts.

Prof G. Appendino

List of Collaborators

S Togni

R Luzzi

L Pellegrini

A Ledda

B Feragalli

M Corsi

E Ippolito

S Hu

M Dugall

U Cornelli

G Gizzi

MR Cesarone

A Saggino

C Gizzi

P Peterzan

M Hosoi

E Bombardelli

Contents

Pharma-Standard Supplements

Introduction

Dietary supplements are the most commonly used of all complementary and 'alternative' treatments. The meaning of alternative and complementary is basically wrong and misleading. Medicine is medicine and these products are well within the boundaries of medicine. The two adjectives have been used and are still used by big pharma operators to decrease their possible value and image in comparison with 'patented' products.

Pharma-standard (PS) supplements are generally safe and widely available — usually without prescriptions — and can be usually obtained without consulting a physician. However, the first indication to the use of supplements should be based on clinical grounds and upon the suggestions of a physician. The Food and Drug Administration (FDA) regulates supplements differently from drugs. Quality control and good manufacturing processes are monitored but the FDA does not define or ensure standardization of the active ingredients or efficacy. Safety issue are always considered as the first issue and most supplements available in the market can be defined as safe.

Definition

The Dietary Supplement Health Education Act (DSHEA) of 1994, defines a dietary supplement as:

"Any product (excluding tobacco and its derivates) — in pill, capsule, tablet or liquid form — containing vitamins, mineral, herb or product derived from plants, amino acid, or other known dietary substance that is intended as a supplement to the normal diet."

Certain hormones, such as dehydroepiandrosterone (DHEA, a precursor to androgens and estrogens) and melatonin, are also regulated as

1

dietary supplements and not as prescription drugs. However, different countries may have different regulations.

Labelling

The DSHEA requires that the product label must clearly identify the product as a dietary supplement; the label should notify the possible consumer that the suggested 'claims' for the supplement have not been evaluated by the FDA.

The label usually includes a list of the ingredients, indicating them by name, indicating their quantity and weight. The label must also identify plant elements from which the ingredients are derived.

Manufacturers are permitted to make some claims about the product's structure and function (e.g., good for urinary tract health) but cannot make or imply specific claims for the product as it is not considered a drug and cannot be considered a specific therapy (e.g., treats UTIs).

Safety and Efficacy

People who use dietary supplements (defined in this volume as *supplements*) have indications suggesting that the supplements are good for health problems and are generally safe. Supplements are considered effective for treating specific risk conditions or preclinical and even clinical conditions.

Most dietary supplements are natural (i.e., they are derived from plant elements) and their history is often supported by centuries of use in traditional systems of medicine.

The FDA does not require manufacturers of supplements to prove their safety or efficacy (generally, supplements must have a long history of safety).

Usually the extraction of the supplements from plants or other sources should be without chemical or solvents that may interfere with the structure and potential toxicity of the products.

Most supplements have not been rigorously, clinically studied (according to big pharma rules). The absence of patents for most supplements, the negative influence of 'big pharma', and the relatively low profits make expensive clinical trials difficult.

For most supplements, evidence suggesting safety or efficacy comes from their traditional use, *in vitro* studies, some case reports and animal studies.

However, manufacturers and distributors of supplements, must report serious adverse side-effects and tolerability problems to the FDA through the MedWatch system.

Some supplements (e.g., fish oil, chondroitin-glucosamine, saw palmetto) have proved to be safe in large and long studies and are considered useful complements to standard treatments and drugs.

Evidence concerning the safety and efficacy of supplements is increasing rapidly as more and more clinical studies are being completed. Most information about these studies is available at the National Institutes of Health's National Center for Complementary and Alternative Medicine (NCCAM) web site (www.nccam.nih.gov/research/clinicaltrials/).

Most important papers are published in peer review journals and quoted in Medline–Pubmed and the most important databases.

However, the specificity of the supplement (unless there are standards) make each supplement formulation different from another. Therefore studies valid for one product cannot be applied to all products derived from the same source.

In this volume we discuss only **PS** supplements that, at least within that specific product formulation, have constant, defined standards, dosages and preventive or therapeutic schemes, clearly defined by clinical studies.

PS supplements have specific formulations (i.e., defined by chromatography), bioavailability and distribution data assessed in human contexts, both in healthy subjects and patients.

Purity and Standardization

Limited regulation and monitoring also means that all supplements are not monitored externally to ensure that they contain the ingredients or amount of active ingredients the manufacturer claims they contain. But most producers monitor the quantity and quality of their products.

The supplement, if not carefully produced and tested, may also have unlisted ingredients which may be inert or even harmful (e.g., natural toxins, bacteria, pesticides, lead or other heavy metals). Supplements may contain variable amounts of active ingredients, especially when whole plant-derived products are ground or made into extracts. However this is a 'moral' and technical issue for the producer and most high quality products (i.e., by blending different extracts, from different years) may always keep the same standards within very narrow limits. It is in the care of the user to consider the quality of the products and its standards. With low-quality products consumers may be at risk of getting less, more, or in some cases, none of the active ingredients.

Most plant-derived supplements include several complex compounds and substances. Which ingredient is the most active or effective is not always known and often the total complex is effective by producing a number of pathways and interactions.

If there is a lack of standardization (it does not happen with high quality products that we define PS), not only products from different producers and manufacturers may vary, but it is also possible that different batches produced by the same manufacturer may differ.

Product variability is a source of technical problems in production; conducting rigorous scientific trials and comparing the results among different trials becomes difficult.

However, some supplements have been standardized at pharma level and may include indications explaining the type of standardization on the label.

Relatively recent regulations governing the production and marketing of supplements in the US include rules for good manufacturing practices (GMPs) that improve and strengthen standards for maintaining manufacturing facilities, equipment clean, and raw materials pure and uncontaminated.

GMPs also ensure proper labeling, packaging and storage of the finished product.

Other Improvements in Supplements and Their Use

Additional areas of improvements in the use of PS supplement in preventive and clinical medical applications may include:

1. The **definition of the correct use** of PS supplements when possible (i.e., in period of remission a supplement could be used instead of standard drug treatment that may be more expensive, may cause more

side effects and may be interactive with other treatments used at the same time).

2. The stability of PS supplements (particularly those derived from *plants*) once manufactured.

   Specific blending procedures may be needed. The quantity and relative compositions of elements in a plant extract are variable every year due to rain, sun and climatic factors.

   To keep a reasonable standard that includes defined ranges of the active compounds an appropriate blending (including compounds from several years) is usually needed and it is a major skill in the preparation of PS supplements.

3. The reduction in possible toxicity as single products and in connection with other acute or chronic treatments the patient may be using (i.e., anticoagulant treatment).

   Relative toxicity, considering special situations (i.e., renal or heart failure), should also be considered.

4. The possible (positive or negative) interactions between PS supplements and 'standard' drugs should be possibly defined for each type of patient and clinical situation.

At the moment most information about significant interactions or negative effects derive from experience reported in sporadic, individual reports and some referenced case reports.

However, many physicians, healthcare operators and patients believe and have experienced the benefit of non-standard and PS supplements.

Patients (and subjects with a risk condition) often use supplements with or without physician's suggestions or involvement.

In some cases, patients may not inform physicians if they use supplements or may conceal their use for several reasons.

Therefore any outpatient history should specifically, clearly, and periodically include explicit questions about the use of supplements (and of any complementary or alternative therapies, including dietary and nutritional supplements).

Now, most physicians include some supplement use into their management and practice.

Reasons include proven benefits of the supplement, a need to control and limit the use of 'standard drug' treatments, the desire to ensure that supplements are used safely and on the basis of defined rules by patients (who may use supplements anyway).

Also many physicians believe (according to scientific considerations and experience) that supplements (particularly PS supplements) are safe and effective.

Often, there are limited results and information to guide patients when considering safety and professional advice is essential.

Many patients may consider that overdoses or overuse will not have negative effects if the supplement is categorized as 'safe'.

The overall number of problems due to dietary supplements is generally limited when considering the overall number of doses taken and that the supplement, if correctly manufactured, and used according to rules, in the right conditions, is generally safe.

Quality is essential. It is important to purchase all PS supplements from a well-known, high quality producer i.e., it has been recommended to buy supplements made in Germany or in Switzerland because in these countries they are generally regulated as drugs and thus the preparations and standards are superior, stricter than in the US or in the Far East.

Generally, low cost, bad packaging, lack of precise information about the compounds, and lack of clear instructions indicate bad quality.

Buying supplements from internet shops may also be a problem and it is better to use well-known brands, producers and retailers.

The following supplements are widely used and are quite popular. They are generally considered effective, and have a list of medical references and particularly indications about their safety.

The safety of supplements in animals (and animal studies) do not mean very much.

Most plants and fruits that animals use would kill us in minutes and many vegetal elements that we use may be dangerous to different animals. We have very different absorption systems and enzymes.

More complete information concerning each supplement is generally available through the NCCAM web site (www.nccam.nih.gov/).

Medline–Pubmed is the real professional key to get all the needed information but the database is mostly for expert evaluation. Patients should not use supplements without some knowledge.

Part 1 — Common Pharma-Standard Supplements

Beanblock

This is a dry extract of *Phaseolus vulgaris* characterized by a standardized composition in alpha amylase inhibitor with inhibiting activity of 1,400 units/mg and phytohaemagglutinin (haemagglutinating activity equal to 16 haemagglutinating units/mg).

This pharma-standard (PS) supplement has shown efficacy in controlling weight in overweight subjects (otherwise healthy individuals) and in helping in different overeating models.

It could be a natural, alternative or a supplementary measure to other weight control products.

Beanblock is generally used an appetite regulator (but appetite is difficult to quantify) and a 'control system' to decrease sugar and high calorie foods absorption. New studies are in progress. No significant side effects have been observed (see Figure 1).

Black Cohosh (*Actaea racemosa*)

Black cohosh is the underground stem of a plant. Native Americans used black cohosh to treat gynecological symptoms and other disorders, including sore throat, kidney problems and depression.

The extract is standardized to contain a well-defined quantity of triterpenes.

Black cohosh does not contain significant amounts of phytoestrogens that can explain its estrogen-like effects, but it contains small amounts of anti-inflammatory compounds, including salicylic acid.

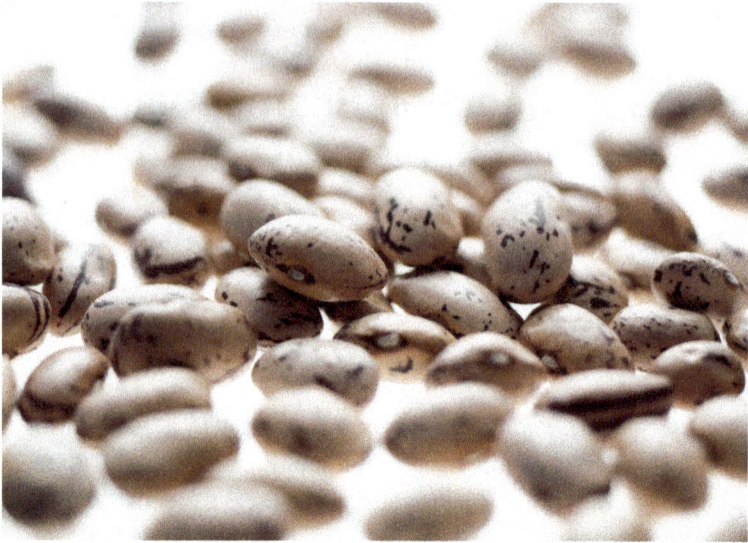

Fig. 1. Beanblock derive from beans

PS supplements of Black cohosh are considered useful for menopausal symptoms and menopausal transition (hot flushes, mood changes, tachycardia, vaginal dryness) for some menstrual symptoms and they have been used for joint pain, arthralgias in rheumatoid arthritis (RA) or osteoarthritis (OA).

Evidence regarding benefits in controlling menstrual symptoms is conflicting, but the effects may be very individual. Patients may try the supplement and, if they find a benefit, they may avoid more complex, prescription drugs that may produce some side effects.

A recent meta-analysis (but this type of evaluation is very inconclusive for supplements from different producers) supports these claims. Study design, clinical targets, dosages, and pharmaceutical characteristics of black cohosh preparations define clinical outcomes.

Some recent clinical investigations with PS supplements indicate that these supplements have some beneficial effects on the physiological pathways underlying age-related disorders like osteoporosis.

Some other recent findings suggest that a part of the clinically relevant effects of black cohosh supplements may be due to compounds that bind and activate serotonin receptors.

A derivative from serotonin with high affinity to serotonin receptors (*N*-methylserotonin) has been identified in black cohosh.

Other complex molecules (including triterpeneglycosides, cycloartanes) have been shown to be effective in reducing cytokine-induced bone loss (osteoporosis) by blocking osteoclastogenesis.

23-*O*-acetylshengmanol-3-*O*-β-D-xylopyranoside, a cycloartane glycoside from *A. racemosa*, has been identified as a modulator of gamma-aminobutyric acid (GABA) receptors with significant sedative activity.

Adverse effects are uncommon (headache and gastrointestinal (GI) problems). Dizziness, diaphoresis and hypotension (only with high dosages) have been reported.

PS supplements from black cohosh do not interfere with any drugs as far as we know. Theoretically, black cohosh supplements are contraindicated in patients with aspirin intolerance, liver disease, hormone-sensitive cancers (breast cancer), stroke or high blood pressure (BP).

The US Pharmacopeia (USP) recommends that black cohosh supplements should be labeled with a warning declaring that they may be hepatotoxic.

Long-term use of black cohosh may cause thickening of the womb possibly leading to an increased risk of womb cancer.

Studies on women using black cohosh preparations did not detect estrogenic effects on the breast (see Figure 2).

Boswellia

Boswellia serrata has a long story of medical applications; it has also been developed for many applications, including topical use.

PS supplements from *B. serrata* include boswellic acid and other pentacyclic triterpene acids. Beta-boswellic acid is considered the major constituent in the extract and supplements.

Boswellia supplements decrease polymorphonuclear leukocyte infiltration and migration, modulate or decrease antibody synthesis and the anticorpal response. The extract almost totally inhibits the classical complement pathway.

PS supplements of boswellia have a potent analgesic and anti-inflammatory activity that controls and reduces the pain and inflammation of joints in patients with arthrosis.

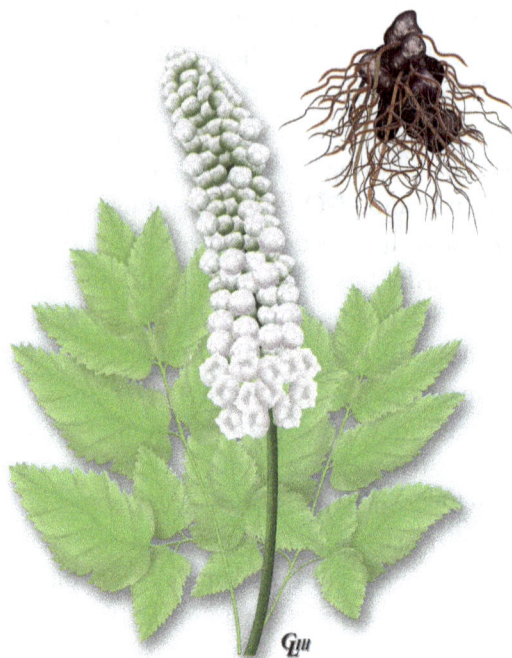

Fig. 2.   Black Cohosh

Boswellia PS supplements and boswellia extracts have been used for the primary or supplementary management of OA and several other inflammatory conditions with significant clinical results.

In these studies, even with different dosages and preparations, boswellia has shown a very good level of tolerability and safety.

A recent Boswellia preparation (a standardized phytoextract from the bark of *B. Serrata*) includes essential oils, gums and terpenoids from boswellic acid.

The standardization process ensures higher bioavailability and efficacy. Its anti-inflammatory efficacy is broadly comparable to non-steroidal anti-inflammatory drugs (NSAID). Boswellia extracts inhibit some proinflammatory mediators such as s-Lipoxygenase and leukotrienes.

New, purified PS supplements and extracts of boswellia do not cause side effects (particularly GI ulcerative complications) and are more active in comparison with other previously available boswellia products. The effects of boswellia PS supplements appear to persist longer (particularly in subjects with significant knee degeneration) and appear to be more effective than other products used to manage OA (i.e., those including chondroitin or glucosamine ($C_6H_{13}NO_5$)). The supplement seems to act rapidly and in a larger and wider number of patients. This compound can be now considered as an effective, important, supplementary treatment in OA patients, particularly in 'remission' phases or when signs/symptoms are reduced or minimal. Boswellia supplements are also very safe (larger safety studies are in progress) and can be specifically used for self-medication.

Other applications showing positive effects of boswellia PS supplements include the improvement of deteriorated cognitive functions and some chronic inflammatory diseases (including RA, bronchial asthma, ulcerative colitis and Crohn's disease).

Several studies have been recently published and there are more studies in progress (see Figure 3).

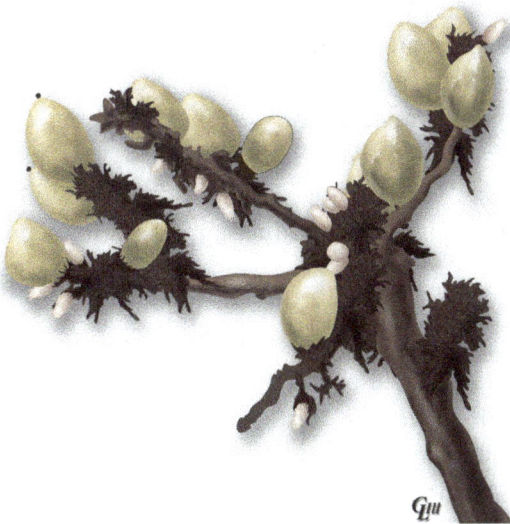

Fig. 3. Boswellia

Centella asiatica (CA)

CA (formerly known as *Hydrocotyle asiatica, also known as Centella o Gotu kola*) is a member of the parsley family. It is native to India, Madagascar, Sri Lanka, Africa, Australia, China and Indonesia.

CA is a small, herbaceous, annual plant of the family Mackinlayaceae or subfamily Mackinlayoideae of family Apiaceae. CA has a long history of use.

It has been used medicinally since 2000 AD even to treat leprosy, to treat wounds and gonorrhea and to treat fever and respiratory infections in China.

CA has large amounts of pentacyclic triterpenoids including asiaticoside, brahmoside, asiatic acid and brahmic acid also known as madecassic acid. Other products include centellose, centelloside, and madecassoside.

The most common use of CA in PS supplements in the United States is in the supplementary treatment for varicose veins and chronic venous insufficiency (CVI).

Several studies using CA in the management of CVI with leg swelling, varicose veins, pain, itching, atrophic skin changes and ulcers and in patients with post-thrombotic limbs have indicated significant improvements in signs and symptoms. CVI has also been evaluated in several prolonged studies, also involving the microcirculation.

Results from these microcirculatory studies suggest that CA and its supplements produce moderate but significant benefits on objective and subjective parameters associated with CVI.

Supplements of CA also appear to promote wound healing (venous ulcers) possibly through the modulation and stimulation of collagen synthesis.

The modulation of collagen is a very important aspect of CA and PS supplements. Too much collagen causes the formation of cheloids (i.e., after burns), particularly in children and may cause an abnormal growth in venous ulcerations, leading to irregular scarring and delayed healing.

Finally, an abnormal accumulation of collagen causes the irregular growth and progression of atherosclerotic plaques. A recent study based on long-term clinical evaluation indicate that the use of a CA PS supplement (in association with Pycnogenol) is effective in modulating the growth of atherosclerotic plaques in carotid and femoral arteries.

Independently from risk factor control, the plaques grow less and slower, and plaque progression is generally delayed. Also, the passage from asymptomatic to symptomatic stages is delayed in most patients with >50% stenosis plaques.

Safety: The FDA does not strictly regulate CA supplements or TTFCA as the other PS supplements. Theoretically, Centella and TTFCA may cause an increase in drowsiness caused by sedatives (i.e., benzodiazepines such as lorazepam, barbiturates, codeine) and interact with alcohol. Caution is advised when driving or using machinery.

Side effects: Minor effects can be observed including stomach upset and nausea. They are very uncommon. CA PS extracts should come from specific and safe plantations. CA grows wildly along ditches and in low, wet areas.

The plant frequently suffers from high levels of bacterial and metal contamination, possibly from having been harvested from sewage ditches or close to contaminated water. Because the plant is aquatic, it is especially sensitive to pollutants in the water, which are easily incorporated into the plant. Low-cost products may be at risk of such contaminations.

Apparently, the plant produced in Madagascar is more effective than comparable plants from other regions particularly in modulating collagen genesis and remodeling (see Figure 4).

Chamomile

The flower of chamomile is dried and used in infusion as tea or used topically as an extract.

Claims: Chamomile may reduce fever and inflammation, it acts as a mild sedative, may relieve stomach cramps and indigestion and it has been used to promote healing of gastric ulcers.

An essential oil including bisabolol is the main constituent. Bisabolol has a weak floral aroma used in fragrances. It has been used in cosmetics for its skin healing effects. Bisabolol is an anti-irritant, anti-inflammatory and antimicrobial agent. It enhances the percutaneous absorption of some molecules. α-bisabolol has been shown to produce apoptosis in models of leukemia.

Chamomile extracts may increase the effects of some anticoagulants and some sedatives (including alcohol) and could decrease the absorption of iron supplements.

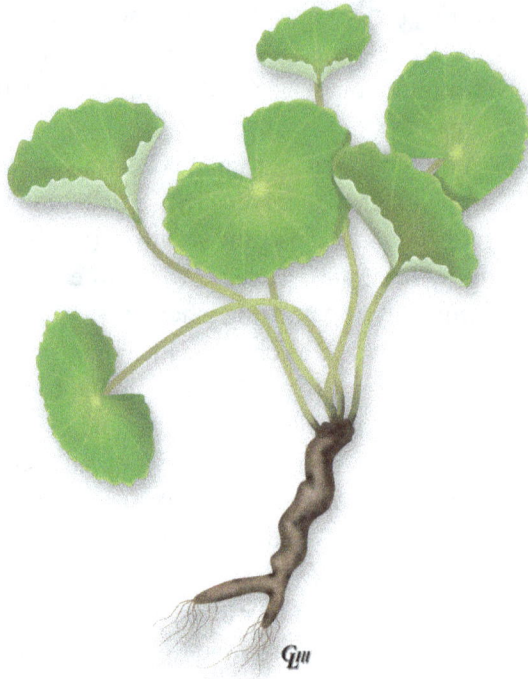

Fig. 4. *Centella Asiatica*

PS supplements are still difficult to find as the traditional use by infusion is very common.

Most present uses include the use of the flower or full flower extracts (see Figure 5).

Chromium

Chromium (Cr) is a trace mineral that potentiates the action of insulin. Nutritional sources of Cr include carrots, potatoes, broccoli and whole grains.

Picolinate (a by-product of tryptophan) is associated with Cr in some PS supplements as there are clinical indications that the complex may help in the absorption of Cr more efficiently.

Cr picolinate may promote — according to several reports — weight loss, build muscle, reduce body fat, lower cholesterol and triglyceride levels and enhance insulin function.

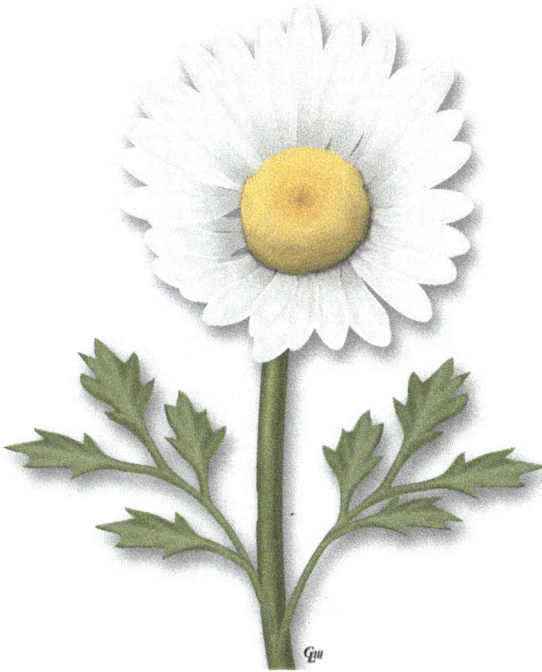

Fig. 5. Chamomile

Cr deficiency impairs insulin function, but there is no evidence that supplementation with Cr may clinically help patients with diabetes.

Adverse effects: Cr picolinate may damage chromosomes and may be a concause of cancer. Some supplements with Cr may cause or contribute to GI irritation and ulcers. Cr supplements interfere with iron absorption. The popular dietary supplement Cr picolinate complex causes chromosome damage (this has been shown in hamster cells due to the picolinate ligand).

In USA, the dietary guidelines for daily chromium uptake were lowered in 2001 from 50 to 200 μg for an adult to 35 μg (adult male) and to 25 μg (adult female).

No comprehensive, reliable database of chromium content of food currently exists. Cr content of food varies widely due to differences in soil mineral content, growing season, plant environment and contamination during processing.

Large amounts of Cr (and nickel) may end into food cooked in stainless steel.

At the moment, basically there is no defined medical use as a supplement and there is no real PS supplement.

Coenzyme Q10

Ubiquinone, ubidecarenone, coenzyme Q or **CoQ10** is a 1,4-benzoquinone: **Q** refers to the quinone group and **10** refers to the number of isoprenyl subunits in its tail.

This oil-soluble, vitamin-like substance is present in most cells, primarily in the mitochondria.

It is associated to the electron transport chain and participates in aerobic cellular respiration, generating energy in the form of adenosine triphosphate (ATP).

In humans, 95% of energy is generated this way. Organs with the highest energy requirements — heart, liver and kidney — have the highest CoQ_{10} concentrations.

There are three redox states of CoQ_{10}: fully oxidized (ubiquinone), semiquinone (ubisemiquinone) and fully reduced (ubiquinol).

The capacity of this molecule to exist in a completely oxidized form and a completely reduced form enables it to perform its functions in the electron transport chain or as an antioxidant.

Coenzyme Q10 (ubiquinone) is a powerful and common antioxidant and a cofactor for mitochondrial ATP generation.

The reduced form of CoQ regenerates Vitamin E from the α-tocopheroxyl radical, interfering with the propagation step.

During oxidative stress, interaction of H_2O_2 with metal ions bound to deoxyribonucleic acid (DNA) generates hydroxyl radicals, and CoQ10 efficiently prevents the oxidation of bases, particularly, in mitochondrial DNA.

In contrast to other antioxidants, this compound inhibits both the initiation and the propagation of lipid and protein oxidation.

It also regenerates other antioxidants such as Vitamin E. The circulating CoQ10 in low-density lipoprotein (LDL) prevents oxidation of LDL, which may provide benefit in cardiovascular diseases.

The levels of coenzyme Q10 are lower in older people and in people with chronic diseases (i.e., chronic cardiac problems, cancer, Parkinson's disease, diabetes, HIV/AIDS and muscular dystrophies) and in patients using statins.

It is not clear how low levels contribute to these disorders.

Claims: Coenzyme Q10 is considered to be useful because of its antioxidant effect and role in energy metabolism.

Specific claims include an anticancer effect mediated by immune stimulation (only weak indications in *in vitro* cellular studies), decreased insulin requirements in patients with diabetes, slowed progression of Parkinson's disease, efficacy in treatment of heart failure and protection against some types of cardiotoxicity.

Although some preliminary studies suggest coenzyme Q10 may be useful in improving or co-treating these disorders, results are not clear and more studies are needed. Supplementation of CoQ_{10} has been found to have a variable effect on migraine.

Adverse effects: Coenzyme Q10 may decrease response to warfarin. There are case reports of GI symptoms (including loss of appetite, abdominal pain, nausea, vomiting) and neurological central nervous system (CNS) symptoms (dizziness, headache, tinnitus, photophobia, irritability) at higher doses.

Other significant adverse effects include itching, rash, fatigue and flu-like symptoms.

Coenzyme Q10 is not generally indicated for people who exercise vigorously.

The common use of statins to treat high lipids to prevent atherosclerosis reduces the levels of CoQ10 and may even cause heart failure in some patients, particularly when ACE inhibitors and CoQ10 are used together.

Supplementation with CoQ10 supplements may restore the levels of CoQ10 in the myocardium and improve ventricular function.

Inhibition by statins and beta blockers: CoQ10 shares a biosynthetic pathway with cholesterol. The synthesis of an intermediary precursor of CoQ10, mevalonate, is inhibited by some beta blockers, BP drugs and by statins (cholesterol-lowering drugs). Statins can reduce serum levels of CoQ10 by up to 40%. Supplementation with CoQ10 may be considered in any treatment — particularly chronic treatments — that may reduce endogenous production of CoQ10.

Colostrum

Colostrum is a milky fluid that comes from the breasts of humans, cows and other mammals the first few days after giving birth before true milk appears.

It contains proteins, carbohydrates, fats, vitamins, minerals and immuno-proteins (antibodies) that fight most common disease causing agents such as bacteria and viruses. Antibody levels in colostrums can be 100 times higher than levels in regular cow's milk.

Colostrum is a GI tract antioxidant and an important aid in the prevention and treatment of problems linked to asthenia, lack of appetite, anemia, pathological conditions, convalescence and metabolic disorders.

Colostrum initially starts the nutrition of the newborn for the first few days of life and at the same time protects the child from the potential aggression of the outside environment at a moment of great vulnerability for the organism.

The intestinal contact surface is a very large, possible site of lethal contamination in babies before they have the protective effect of their immunoglobulins.

Colostrum is considered as the 'first vaccination' considering the large number of antibodies it contains.

Among the most vulnerable parts of the newborns, the GI tract is very vulnerable for a few days after birth.

The vulnerability does not completely disappear after the first few days of life and may lead to several problems and disorders, sometimes limited to unpleasant symptoms and sometimes leading to acute or chronic diseases. A large number of diseases has its origin in the intestinal tract.

Intestinal dysbiosis identifies a condition of reduced intestinal defensive function with immunologic, inflammatory and infective problems. Colostrum restores the GI environment and as a consequence, systemic health particularly in newborns but also in adults.

Proline-rich polypeptides (PRP) have been discovered in colostrum (they are present in blood plasma). These polypeptides have been named

Colostrinin, CLN, transfer factor and PRP. They function as signal transducing molecules that have the unique effect of modulating the immune system, turning it up when the body comes under attack from pathogens or other disease agents, and damping it when the danger is eliminated or neutralized. At first thought to transfer immunity from one immune system to another, it now appears that PRP stimulates cell-mediated immunity.

PS colostrum has been used to prevent infectious and viral episodes. A recent study indicated that colostrum as PS supplement can be used for the prevention of flu and cold in otherwise healthy subjects.

Colostrum was superior (in preventing viral and flu episodes) to flu vaccination both in healthy and high-risk cardiovascular subjects and subjects with pulmonary disease.

Colostrum was also useful to prevent a number of hospital admissions and moderate to severe complications in older subjects.

Colostrum is indicated in improving weakness (i.e., after convalescence) in elderly people to prevent flu and infections and in weaker people. It has also been used and abused by unsporty athletes or muscle exhibitionists: the effects are questionable and in association with metabolic steroids may theoretically promote cancer.

However, bovine colostrum is not on the banned drug list of the International Olympic Committee.

Adverse effects: No significant side effects have been reported. Subject allergic to cow's milk or milk products may also be allergic to bovine colostrum.

In this condition, it is best to avoid colostrum supplementation.

Condroitin Sulfate

Condroitin sulphate (CS) is a sulfated glycosaminoglycan (GAG) composed of a chain of alternating sugars (*N*-acetylgalactosamine and glucuronic acid). It is usually found attached to proteins as part of a proteoglycan. A chondroitin chain may have over 100 individual sugars, each of which can be sulfated in variable positions and quantities. Chondroitin sulfate is an important structural component of cartilage and is an essential component for its resistance to compression. CS is considered an essential, natural component of any healthy cartilage. It is generally extracted to produce supplements from shark or cow cartilage. It can also be produced synthetically. It is often combined for clinical applications with $C_6H_{13}NO_5$.

CS is used to manage OA and its signs/symptoms. In combination with $C_6H_{13}NO_5$, CS reduces joint pain, and improves joint mobility; these effects allow a significant reduction of the doses of conventional anti-inflammatory drugs and corticosteroids. The effects on symptoms are generally seen after 6–24 months of treatment.

Structural effects on the joints are seen over longer periods but appear unclear.

The dose is generally around 600 mg (*per os*) once daily or 400 mg, three times daily.

No serious adverse effects have been seen considering that products including CS are widely used by a large number of patients for long periods.

CS is a prescription or over-the-counter drug in 22 countries but is regulated in the US as a dietary supplement by the FDA. In Europe, most CS formulations are approved as drugs with evidence of efficacy and safety shown in clinical trials in OA patients.

Common adverse effects are stomach pain, nausea and GI symptoms.

CS may affect the activity of the anticoagulant warfarin.

Adverse effects: Products including CS are generally considered safe, but people with asthma, blood-clotting disorders or prostate cancer should use CS with some caution when taking it or consider alternatives.

Cranberry

In Britain, cranberry may refer to the native species *Vaccinium oxycoccos*, while in North America, cranberry may refer to *Vaccinium macrocarpon*. Cranberries are fruits that are usually consumed fresh or dried, made into food products (jellies, juices), extracts and PS supplements.

Claims: PS cranberry supplements help to prevent and relieve the symptoms of urinary tract infections (UTIs) and post-infection inflammation. The efficacy of cranberries in preventing UTIs has been shown in several studies. Natural, unprocessed cranberry juice contains anthocyanidins which prevent *Escherichia coli* (*E. coli*) from colonizing the urinary tract wall.

Cranberry juice may reduce fever in some patients.

Problems may arise with the lack of validation of a standard method for the quantification of A-type proanthocyanidins.

In the case of most cranberry extracts, it can be performed using several existing methods including for example, the European Pharmacopoeia method, liquid chromatography–mass spectrometry (LC-MS) or a modified 4-dimethyl-aminocinnamaldehyde (DMAC) colorimetric method. This may lead to difficulties in evaluating the real quality of extracts from different origins.

Studies indicate that quality varies greatly from one commercial Cranberry product to another, but most products are actually, clinically effective.

Cranberry PS supplements are becoming more common and with defined quantity of active substances.

Recent studies in different types of patients indicate that a cranberry PS supplement decreases the number of urinary infection episodes in two months in prone subjects, elder patients with prostatic hypertrophy and younger subjects.

Good results have been obtained in premenopausal women in several studies.

After a UTI due to a specific pathogen (i.e., *E. coli*) and antibiotic treatment, UTI may persist as an inflammation more than an infection. The inflammation at mucosal level may be painful and prolonged. PS cranberry supplements seem to be able to reduce post-infective inflammation without the real need for antibiotic treatment. After any urinary catheterization (i.e., after surgery of urinary procedures), this type of inflammation may be difficult to solve and antibiotics may not be very effective.

PS cranberry, in most of its forms, may help to control signs and symptoms of post-infective, mucosal inflammation.

Adverse effects: No adverse effects are known. However, because most cranberry juices include sugar to offset its tart taste, diabetics should use cranberry juice with some caution, considering potential sugar content and artificial sweeteners.

This problem is not present when using PS supplements in capsules.

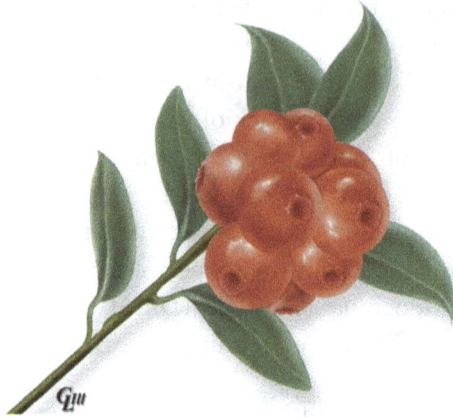

Fig. 6. Cranberry

Cranberry supplements increase urinary acidity and, theoretically, may promote stone formation in patients with story of uric acid kidney stones.

Also, cranberry supplementation may occasionally increase the effects of warfarin (see Figure 6).

Creatine

Creatine is a nitrogenous organic acid present naturally in all vertebrates that helps to supply energy to all cells and primarily to muscle cells. This effect is achieved by increasing the formation of ATP.

Phosphocreatine is stored in the human muscle. This compound donates phosphate to ADP and rapidly replenishes ATP during periods of anaerobic muscle contraction.

Creatine is synthesized endogenously in the liver from arginine, glycine and methionine.

It is generally found in milk, meat and some fish. Creatine may help to improve physical and athletic performance also reducing muscular fatigue.

This element has been found effective at increasing the efficiency of exercise in short maximal efforts (sprinting, weightlifting).

Creatine has a defined therapeutic use in muscle phosphorylase deficiency (glycogen storage disease type V or McArdle disease) and gyrate atrophy of the choroid and retina.

Some clinical studies indicate some possible, positive effects in Parkinson's disease and amyotrophic lateral sclerosis.

Improved cognitive ability: A prospective study found that vegetarians/ vegans who took 5 g of creatine per day (six weeks) showed a significant improvement on two tests of fluid intelligence. This study indicated that supplementation with creatine significantly increased attention and 'intelligence' considering that evaluation methods and tests are often questionable in this field.

Other studies found that creatine PS supplements improved some cognitive ability in elderly subjects. Why this action should be produced by creatine is still unclear, but studies are in progress.

Adverse effects: Creatine may cause weight gain (possibly because of an increase in muscle mass) and increases in serum creatinine. Minor GI symptoms, dehydration, electrolytic imbalance and muscle cramps have been reported.

Pregnancy and breastfeeding: There is no clear scientific information on the effects of creatine supplementation during pregnancy and breastfeeding. It is not clear if taking creatine during pregnancy affects the rate of cerebral palsy or other neurological problems. Pasteurized cow's milk contains higher levels of creatine than human milk.

Curcumin

Curcumin is the yellow pigment of turmeric (*Curcuma longa*), the most popular spice in Indian cuisine, a major ingredient of curry. The dietary intake of curcumin in Asian countries can reach much as 200 mg/day.

In the UK population, the mean and maximum reported use levels of curcumin have been estimated, combining the use of curcumin from naturally occurring curcumin in foods (turmeric as spice and in curry powder) and from its use as a food color, at over 50 mg/day and 210 mg/day, respectively, in the adult population.

Turmeric has a long history of medicinal use in India to control or treat many conditions.

Cellular studies on curcumin have validated most of its traditional uses and have indicated its old and new potentials to control some risk conditions and diseases.

With some 4,000 preclinical investigations, curcumin is one of the best studied and known natural products within the biomedical field.

Literature: Curcumin has recently emerged as a significant, important compound to control and treat natural and abnormal inflammatory responses. Its actions include both a direct and a genomic activity on relevant enzymes, action on transcription factors and on cytokines.

Recent clinical evidence has raised a great interest for curcumin, particularly considering the new PS formulations.

Still, most of the beneficial effects of curcumin are shown or suggested by epidemiological studies.

Animal models — as for most 'natural' supplements — may be interesting but hardly conclusive.

The new PS Supplement curcumin (Meriva®, bioavailable curcumin) is a patented delivery form. Curcumin and soy lecithin are formulated in a 1:2 weight ratio, and two parts of microcrystalline cellulose are then added to improve flowability with an overall content of curcumin in the final product of around 20%. Meriva® is based on Phytosome® technology aimed to improve the bioavailability of compounds like polyphenolics and triterpenoid acids that are normally characterized by poor solubility both in water and in organic solvents.

Curcumin, just like most dietary phenolics, is not very soluble in water or in oily solvents, but shows polar groups that interact via hydrogen bondings and polar interactions with complementary groups, like the polar heads of phospholipids.

Thus, soy lecithin has a highly polarized head with the negative charge of a phosphate group and the positive charge of the choline ammonium group and can complex a variety of poorly soluble phenolics including curcumin.

Phenolics as curcumin, show a high affinity for biological membranes and, once complexed with phospholipids, are embedded into a lipidic matrix that can capitalize on the rapid exchange of phospholipids between biological membranes and the extracellular fluids, shuttling it into biological membranes. This mechanism increases its cellular captation to significant levels, improving its clinical characteristics.

Studies on Meriva® (complexed curumin) have addressed the natural and abnormal inflammatory response processes.

The use of curcumin for bone health is based on the capacity of this compound to interrupt most inflammatory response signaling and increases antioxidant levels.

Evidence indicate that bone/joint health is better supported by agents that modulate multiple cellular targets and curcumin has a great potential for the management of these conditions.

Curcumin (particularly the new formulation Meriva®) has shown its efficacy in individuals with knee arthrosis.

Their symptoms (evaluated by the WOMAC score), mobility (studied by walking performance on a treadmill) and the overall inflammatory response function (C-reactive protein) improved in three months using curcumin (between 1 and 2 g/day).

The treadmill walking test, particularly, indicated a significant improvement in walking. Also, subjects using curcumin used less 'standard' treatments and managements with a significant reduction in costs.

Recent studies on visual impairment also indicated a significant action of curcumin in subjects with diabetic microangiopathy.

Other studies showed the effects on peripheral microcirculation in diabetic microangiopathy, on the inflammatory response and a positive effect of curcumin on subjects exercising in sports.

Another important study indicated that curcumin as Meriva® was effective in decreasing unwanted side effects in subjects treated with radio and chemotherapy without changing the global effects of treatments.

Pharmacokinetics studies of curcumin include a broad range of experiences. In accordance with previous studies, using 'standard' curcumin, 99% of this product after oral administration was present in plasma as glucuronides with the remaining 1% being curcumin sulphate and free curcumin.

Formulation with phospholipids led to a marked (over 20-fold) increase in the concentration of plasma curcumin (essentially glucuronides) and for a longer period of time.

Curcumin in conclusion is one of the most studied PS supplements and could be a significant model supplement for other product evaluation.

The observation that subjects and populations using daily quantities of curcumin in their food in some areas of India have a low incidence of

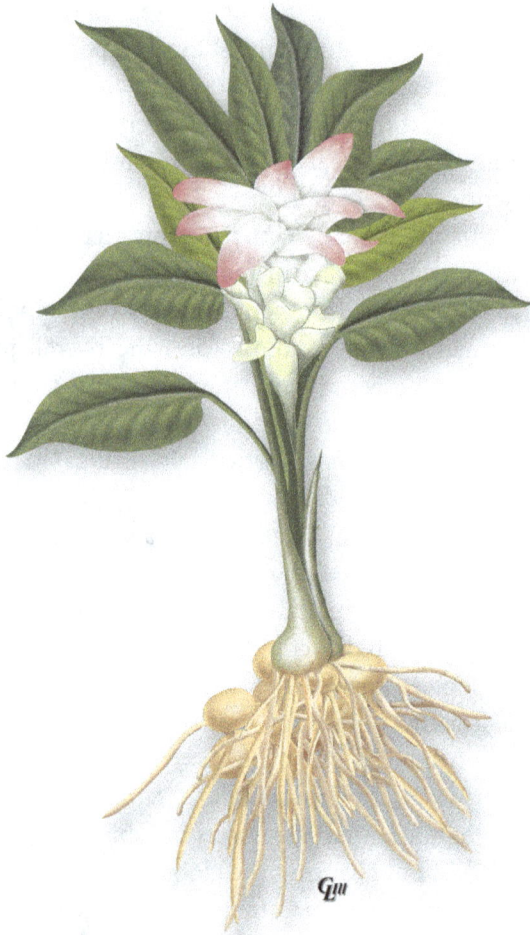

Fig. 7.   Curcuma

cerebral degenerative disease with older age and a lower incidence of prostatic problems may indicate future use of this product.

Ethnopharmacology may identify areas with a lower incidence of a clinical problem and connect the low incidence with some nutritional or environmental elements that may contribute to decrease in the occurrence of some diseases or conditions (see Figure 7).

Dehydroepiandrosterone

Dehydroepiandrosterone (DHEA) more correctly diDHEA, also known as androstenolone or prasterone (INN), as well as 3β-hydroxyandrost-5-en-17-one or 5-androsten-3β-ol-17-one, is an important endogenous steroid hormone. This steroid produced by the adrenal gland is a precursor of estrogens and androgens. It is considered a supplement. Its effects are quite similar to those of testosterone. DHEA also has a variety of biological effects, binding to several nuclear and cell surface receptors and acting as a neurosteroid.

DHEA can also be synthesized from precursors in the Mexican yam; this product is the most commonly available.

Claims: In women with adrenal insufficiency and in the healthy elderly subjects, there is very limited evidence supporting the use of DHEA.

These PS supplements have been found to improve mood, energy, sense of well-being, and the ability to perform better under stress.

DHEA may improve athletic performance, stimulate the immune system, deepen night sleep, lower cholesterol levels, decrease body fat, build muscles, improve attention and brain functions in patients with Alzheimer's disease and possibly increase libido.

A bit too much, but actually, the medicinal claims of DHEA are still unproven.

DHEA is sold in the USA as a dietary supplement. It is one of the oldest dietary ingredients (being in the market since 1994). DHEA is exempted from the Anabolic Steroid Control Act, but it is banned from use in athletic competition.

Rashard Lewis (Orlando Magic, NBA) tested positive for DHEA and was suspended 10 games before the start of the 2009–2010 season.

2008 Olympic 400 meter champion Lashawn Merritt also tested positive for DHEA and was banned from events for 21 months.

DHEA and DHEAS are readily available in the United States, where they are marketed as over-the-counter dietary supplements.

DHEA supplements have been considered useful to improve memory functions in normal middle aged or older adults.

DHEA has also been studied as a specific treatment for Alzheimer's disease, but, at the moment, there is no evidence that the product may be effective.

More studies also suggest that low serum levels of DHEAS may be associated with coronary heart disease in men.

At the moment, there is no evidence to indicate whether DHEA supplementation might have any significant cardiovascular action or benefit of the progression of the most common cardiovascular conditions.

Some preliminary evidence indicates a short-term benefit of DHEA in patients with systemic lupus erythematosus. However, there is little evidence of long-term benefits or safety in these patients.

Adverse effects are not well-known and are related to dosages. There are theoretical risks of gynecomastia in men, hirsutism in women and possibly, facilitation or stimulation of prostate and breast cancers.

There are reports of manic symptoms and one of seizure, but it is quite possible that not all side effects have been reported.

DHEA is possibly non-safe to use in subjects with possible pregnancy and breastfeeding, in hormone-sensitive conditions, in liver problems, subjects with diabetes, depression or mood disorders. Also, subjects with polycystic ovarian syndrome (PCOS) or cholesterol problems should avoid DHEA.

Individuals with any of these conditions should consult a doctor before supplementation.

Higher levels of DHEA (as other endogenous sex hormones) are strongly associated with an *increased* risk of developing breast cancer in both pre- and postmenopausal women.

Echinacea

Echinacea is originally a North American wildflower, and contains a variety of biologically active substances. The echinacea genus has nine species of flowers, commonly called **coneflowers**.

Echinacea purpurea is the most commonly used plant to produce medicinal extracts. The echinacea PS products that are marketed and studied in clinical trials may be very different.

The supplements contain different species (*E. purpurea, Echinacea angustifolia, Echinacea pallidia*), different organs (roots and herbs), different preparations (extracts and juice) and definitely have different chemical compositions.

Clinical and registry studies are limited at the moment. The multiple meta-analyses are hopeless, as usual, comparing not apples with oranges but figs with meteorites and have no clinical meaning.

The variability of the echinacea products used in the several studies we may consider is impossibly large.

According to recent studies, common cold may be affected by some echinacea PS products. Echinacea may be used to stimulate the immune system. When taken at the start of a cold, echinacea supplements may shorten the duration of symptoms.

Some topical preparations appear to promote wound healing, but more studies are needed.

Adverse effects are usually mild and transitory (dizziness, fatigue, headache and GI symptoms).

No other significant adverse effects are known.

Echinacea should not be used in patients with autoimmune disorders, multiple sclerosis, AIDS, TB and after organ transplants because it may stimulate T cells.

However, the effects could be minimal and clinically irrelevant.

Echinacea also inhibits some cytochrome P-450 enzymes and stimulates other enzymes; it can therefore interact with some drugs metabolized by the same enzymes (anabolic steroids, azole antifungals, methotrexate). Some allergic reactions are possible in patients with pollen allergies.

The European Herbal Medicinal Products Committee (HMPC) and the UK Herbal Medicines Advisory Committee (HMAC) recommended not to use echinacea-containing products in children under the age of 12. Manufacturers label all oral echinacea products that had product licenses for children with a warning that they should not be given to children under 12.

Pregnancy: No study has found increased risk of birth defects associated with echinacea during the first trimester, but pregnant women should avoid echinacea products (but these women should avoid any other product that is not essential).

Among echinacea PS supplements, Immunoselect® (produced with *E. angustifolia* roots harvested in the US) is standardized to contain at least 4% of echinacoside, the major polyphenols in *E. angustifolia* root.

It includes Isobutylamides with an anti-inflammatory and pain relief action.

E. purpurea extract (≥0.8% of caftaric, chicoric, chlorogenic acids and echinacoside) is also considered a significant immune modulator.

Polinacea® (also an immunomodulator from plants cultivated in Italy) is a standardized extract from the roots of *E. angustifolia.*

These plants guarantee both a very high title on polysaccharide as well as any possible cross-contamination between *Echinacea* species.

The PS supplement contains a high molecular weight polysaccharide (IDN 5405) of ca. 20,000 Da identified for the very first time in the *E. angustifolia* root, specific to this plant that has been standardized to be without isobutylamides (≤0.1%).

The standardization of the many products from the different plants is still in progress. Without standards, the product is not clearly usable from a clinical point of view.

Echinacea may also be very important as a co-supplement in other PS supplements (i.e., in association with Saw palmetto (SP) for prostatic hyperthrophy) (see Figure 8).

Feverfew

Feverfew is a bushy perennial herb. The dried leaves are used in capsules, tablets, and in liquid extracts.

Parthenolides and glycosides are thought to be the components responsible for its known anti-inflammatory effects and for the relaxant effects on smooth muscle.

Claims: Feverfew has been considered to be effective in the prevention of migraine headaches. Evidence from three or four relatively small but good quality studies supports these claims. A larger study, however, does not confirm the activity of this product.

Most of these studies may have very subjective clinical targets.

Differences among study findings may also depend on the different formulations of feverfew used.

Feverfew is also considered to be useful for relieving menstrual pain, asthma, and arthritis.

In *in vitro* studies, feverfew inhibits platelet aggregation.

Adverse effects: Mouth ulcers, contact dermatitis, dysgeusia (a distortion of the sense of taste; **dysgeusia** is often associated with ageusia, the complete lack of taste) and mild GI symptoms have been described.

Abrupt discontinuation may worsen migraines and cause anxiety, nervousness and insomnia. Feverfew supplements are contraindicated in pregnant women. In theory, it is also contraindicated in patients taking other antimigraine drugs, iron supplements, NSAIDs, antiplatelet drugs or warfarin.

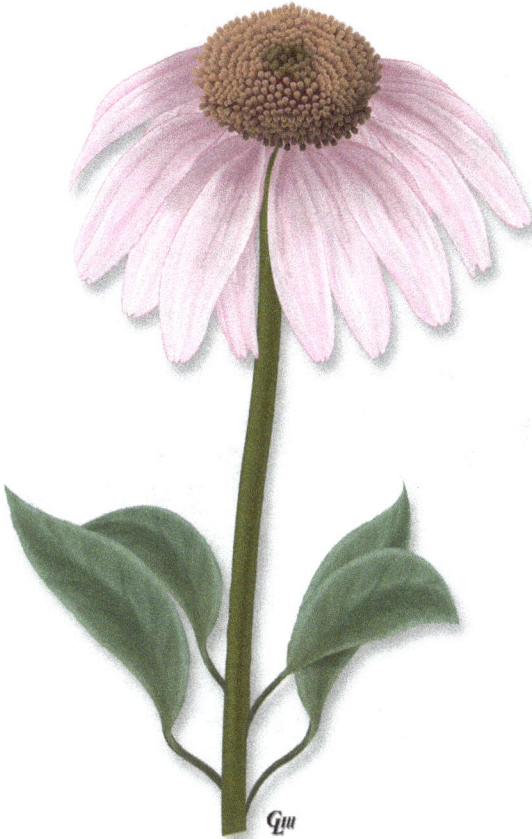

Fig. 8. Coneflower

Ideally, subjects with frequent migraine may try these products and if they have subjective benefits, they may use them for a period as an alternative management to the 'standard' drugs, avoiding a number of side effects (see Figure 9).

Fish Oil

Fish Oil (FO) is one of the best studied supplements. It is generally derived from the tissues of oily fish. FO contain the omega-3 fatty acids, eicosapentaenoic acid (EPA) and docosahexaenoic acid (DHA), precursors of

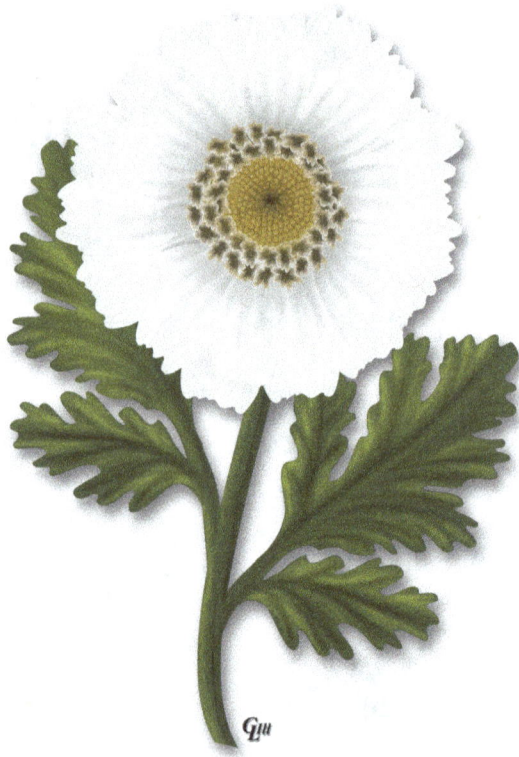

Fig. 9. Feverfew

certain eicosanoids that are known to reduce inflammation in the body and have several other health benefits.

FO may be extracted directly or concentrated and produced in capsules to reach PS.

Main active ingredients are omega-3 fatty acids (EPA and DHA).

Western diets are typically low in omega-3 fatty acids.

Claims: FO supplementation is used for prevention and treatment of atherosclerotic cardiovascular disease and for its complementary management.

There is a long list of studies with strong scientific evidence suggesting that FO supplementation with EPA/DHA (from 80 to 1500 mg daily) reduces the risks of myocardial infarction and death due to arrhythmia in patients with pre-existing coronary artery disease and using 'standard' treatments.

FO also reduces triglycerides and its effects appear to be dose-dependent (25–40% with EPA/DHA 4 g/day).

Most PS supplements of FO tend to slightly lower BP (2–4 mmHg with EPA/DHA >3 g/day).

FO and omega-3 fatty acids have been studied in a variety of other conditions, such as depression, anxiety, oncological conditions, cancer, retinal problems and macular degeneration.

Benefits in these conditions need better evaluation in longer studies involving a large number of patients as in all these preventive studies.

The effects of FO supplementation on prostate hypertrophy or cancer is not clear.

There is a decreased risk with higher blood levels of DHA, but there is an increased risk of a more aggressive prostate cancer with higher blood levels of EPA and DHA in combination.

Some evidence of an association between high blood levels of omega-3 fatty acids, and an increased cancer risk has been observed.

It is clear that a prevention of any cancer may require a long follow up and large study populations.

Alzheimer's disease: A meta-analysis (in June 2012) found no significant protective effect for cognitive decline for those aged 60 and over and who started taking fatty acids after this age. The analysis appears faulty (as most of these analyses, putting together different clinical conditions and different supplements) and suggests that there is no evidence that omega-3 fatty acid supplements provide a benefit for memory or concentration in later life. The target points were very weak and questionable.

However, all these kinds of summary analysis are very questionable and there is not a PS supplement or a therapeutic or preventive protocol for these conditions.

This kind of analysis, often faulty with standard drugs and treatments, is almost impossible for supplements that may have (and usually have) completely different standards and dosages.

Lupus: The disease activity, especially in the skin and joints, was significantly reduced in patients who received FO supplements. There were also changes in the blood platelets of the patients who used the FO supplements.

Inflammatory proteins were also reduced.

Psoriasis: Diets supplemented with cod oil have shown beneficial effects on symptoms of psoriasis in many patients.

FO used during pregnancy may reduce an infant's sensitization to some food allergens reducing frequence and severity of certain skin diseases in the first year of life.

This effect may persist until adolescence with a reduction in prevalence or severity of eczema, hay fever and asthma.

Some national boards and group of specialists recommend a daily intake of 300–500 mg while US do not have recommendation for EPA and DHA.

The American Heart Association recommends 250–500 mg/day of EPA and DHA.

The FDA (USA) recommends not exceeding 3 g/day of EPA and DHA omega-3 fatty acids with no more than 2 g/day from a supplement.

The concentrations of EPA and DHA in PS supplements can vary from 8 to 80% of FO content.

The concentration depends on the source of the omega-3s, how the oil is processed, and the amounts of other ingredients included in the supplement.

Consumers of oily fish should be aware of the potential presence of heavy metals and fat-soluble pollutants like PCBs and dioxins, which are known to accumulate to the food chain particularly in larger fish living longer in the sea. This risk is almost abstent with krill FO.

Researchers from Harvard's School of Public Health in the *Journal of the American Medical Association* (2006) reported that the benefits of fish intake generally far outweigh the potential risks produced by its regular use.

Microalgae oil is a vegetarian alternative to FO. Supplements produced from microalgae oil provide a balance of omega-3 fatty acids similar to FO, with a lower risk of pollutant exposure.

Krill-derived FO is an important alternative and it is generally free of contaminants.

Krill oil also contains naturally occurring Astaxanthin, which has an important antioxidant activity (this product gives krill oil its natural red color).

Garlic

Allium sativum, commonly known as **garlic**, is a species in the onion genus, Allium. The extracts from garlic bulbs are generally produced into tablets. The major active ingredient allicin is an amino acid by-product.

There are two subspecies of *A. sativum*, ten major groups of varieties, hundreds of varieties or cultivars and the supplements have a large variability.

Claims: Garlic is considered to have a number of actions and positive, protective effects on most cardiovascular risk factors (including a mild reduction in BP, lipid and possibly in glucose levels).

The inhibition of platelet aggregation has been documented in *in vitro* studies, but, probably, it does not have a real clinical meaning.

The idea that garlic may protect against laryngeal, gastric, colorectal, endometrial cancers and adenomatous colorectal polyps is almost impossible to prove (or disprove).

No significant evidence is available.

At high doses, garlic has generally mild antimicrobial effects of minimal clinical value.

Believe it or not, the Cochrane group had time to make a meta-analysis on garlic and some researchers have organized clinical trials using garlic. Results are more confusing than the single studies.

Some experiments have been performed on subjects with the common cold, however with limited results.

Adverse effects: Breath and garlicky body smell cannot be considered a real side effect. Occasionally, nausea may occur. High doses may cause burning in the mouth, esophagus, and stomach. In theory, garlic supplements are not indicated in patients who have high risk of bleeding or subjects that use antihypertensives, antiplatelet drugs or anticoagulants.

At the moment, garlic is more a condiment (used to enhance the flavor of foods or to characterize some dishes, particularly in the Mediterranean cuisine) than a real supplement with a clinical meaning.

There is not a single disease that can be affected by garlic supplements.

Ginger

Ginger is extracted from the rhizome of the plant *Zingiber officinale*, traditionally consumed as a delicacy, medicine or spice. Other notable members of this plant family are turmeric, cardamom and galangal.

The distantly related dicots in the Asarum genus have the common name of wild ginger because of their similar taste.

The extracts are generally processed into dosed tablet form and PS supplements.

Active ingredients of ginger include gingerols (which give ginger its flavor and odour) and shogaols.

Claims: Ginger is considered to be an antiemetic and anti-nausea, especially when nausea is caused by motion sickness or pregnancy.

It has been used to relieve intestinal cramps.

Ginger is also used as an anti-inflammatory and analgesic agent.

It may have weak antibacterial properties and antiplatelet effects, but studies are limited.

Several studies indicate a beneficial effect in pregnancy-related nausea and vomiting. Ginger has a sialogogue action, stimulating the production of saliva, which makes swallowing easier and reduces dryness.

According to the American Cancer Society, ginger has been promoted as a cancer prevention tool, but there is no evidence in humans.

A study at the University of Michigan has demonstrated that gingerols can inhibit growth of ovarian cancer cells *in vitro*.

The clinical value of this finding is very relative and cannot be easily translated to clinical contexts.

Ginger PS supplements may significantly affect arthritis pain, lower lipids and particularly cholesterol, but these effects have not been defined in large studies with PS products.

Tea brewed from ginger is considered a common remedy for cold.

PS supplements in the form of gummy caramels have been recently used to promote salivary production keeping the mouth wet.

This effect has a significant activity against cold (the virus appears to spread better on dry mucosal surfaces).

Also, the production of salivary lysozyme may increase up to five times with these gummy ginger caramels and it may be elevated for hours.

Subjects with Bechet's disease (recurrent oral aphthous ulcers, genital ulcers and uveitis) appear to have significant symptomatic benefits (the study is in progress).

Adverse effects: Ginger is usually not harmful, but some people may have a burning sensation when they eat or drink the extracts.

Nausea and dyspepsia have been reported.

In theory, ginger should not be used in patients with bleeding or coagulation problems or treated with anticoagulants or antiplatelet drugs.

Some reports also indicate that ginger may be mutagenic; therefore, the use in pregnant women should be limited particularly in the first trimester (see Figure 10).

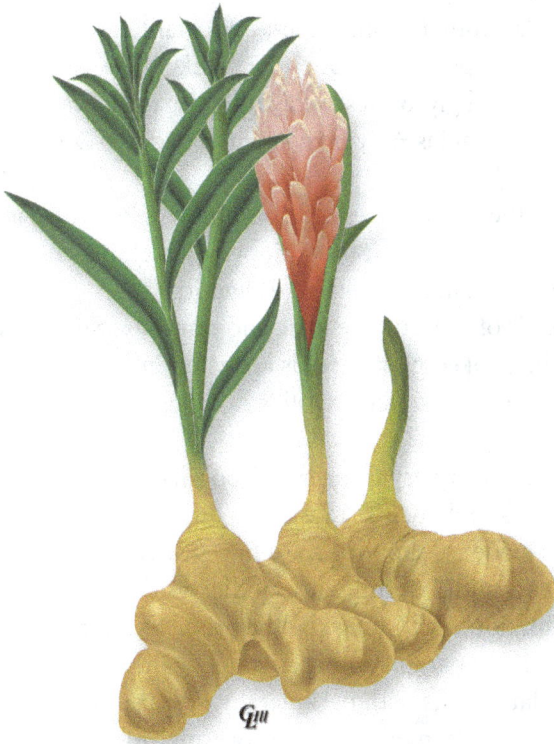

Fig. 10. Zingiber

Ginkgo

Ginkgo biloba (GB) is prepared from leaves of the ginkgo tree (commonly planted in Japan and in the US for ornamental purposes). It is considered a fossil plant: its remnants have been found in fossils from 270 million years.

The plant is extremely resistant; some Ginkgo trees survived the atomic blast in Hiroshima and are still alive.

The ancient Chinese name for *Ginkgo* is yingo or silver fruit. This got changed as *Ginnan* in Japanese but in Kanji characters that can also be pronounced as *Ginkyo*.

Active ingredients are believed to be terpene ginkgolides and flavonoids.

PS extracts of ginkgo leaves contain flavonoid glycosides (myricetin and quercetin) and terpenoids (ginkgolides, bilobalides).

The plant also contains biflavones; important constituents present in the leaves are the terpene trilactones, i.e., ginkgolides A, B, C, J and bilobalide, many flavonol glycosides, biflavones, proanthocyanidins, alkylphenols, simple phenolic acids, 6-hydroxykynurenic acid, 4-O-methylpyridoxine and polyprenols.

The fruit of the gingko tree, which is quite malodorous, is not used in ginkgo products. Contact with the fruit pulp, which may be present under female ginkgo trees, can cause severe dermatitis).

The raw seeds of the fruit are toxic and can cause seizures and, in large amounts, death. Cooked ginkgo seeds are eaten in Asia.

The seeds do not contain ginkgolides and flavonoids; they do not have therapeutic effects.

Claims: There is a very diffuse and popular literature, but the hard evidence with PS supplements is relatively limited.

Some good evidence supports the efficacy of GB in peripheral vascular disease in patients with intermittent claudication.

Supplementation with Ginkgo — the products are generally vasodilating agents, quite comparable to papaverine — increases the walking distance in most claudicants with peripheral vascular diseases.

However standards, management protocols and dosages are not clear and need a full evaluation.

Ginkgo has been used in people with dementia considered to be a consequence of altered flow and microcirculation in the brain.

However, benefits of treatment in dementia are really difficult to show: in a recent clinical trial, ginkgo was not effective in reducing the progression of dementia and Alzheimer's disease in older people. But then nothing is really effective in these conditions.

It is a wrong, impossible model to test a supplement.

Previous US trials indicated that ginkgo supplementation temporarily stabilized mental and social functions in people with mild to moderate dementia. Again, it is a difficult model.

These indications are very controversial and effects may be very marginal. But for many people, there is no real drug alternative or treatments.

Other studies show that supplementation with ginkgo does not seem to alleviate memory loss (at the moment, nothing can!), tinnitus or altitude sickness.

Ginkgo may prevent some damage to the kidneys caused by the immunosuppressant cyclosporine.

Retinal arterial flow can be improved with supplementation. Also, the microcirculation appears to be affected by Ginko supplements, but the clinical efficacy of these microcirculatory effects is not available.

Gingko powder (from dried leaves) appears to improve the healing of some vascular ulcerations (venous and diabetics).

Adverse effects: Nausea, dyspepsia, headache, dizziness, heart palpitations may occur with high dosages in some individuals.

Ginkgo may theoretically interact with aspirin, NSAIDs, antiplatelet agents and anticoagulants (but there is no clear evidence) and may reduce the efficacy of some anticonvulsants. Ginkgo PS supplements may inhibit monoamine oxidase; patients using some antidepressants (such as monoamine oxidase inhibitors (MAOIs) and selective serotonin reuptake inhibitor (SSRI)) may have side effects including an increased risk of developing serotonin syndrome, a life-threatening condition.

There are hundreds of products under the definition of GB, but only PS supplements with clear definition of the products should be considered (see Figure 11).

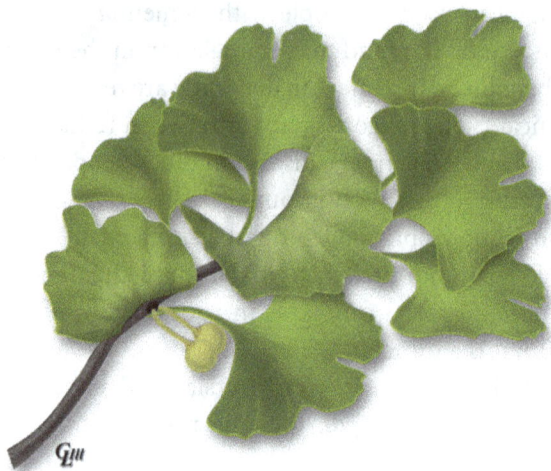

Fig. 11.   Gingko

Ginseng

Ginseng is a family of plants. The term ginseng defines any one of 11 species of slow-growing perennial plants with fleshy roots, part of the genus Panax (family *Araliaceae*). PS supplements of ginseng are mostly derived from the American ginseng (*Panax quinquefolius*) or Asian ginseng. Siberian ginseng is a different genus and does not contain the ingredients believed to be active in the two forms used in supplements.

Ginseng can be used as a fresh product or dried roots, extracts, solutions, capsules, tablets, in sodas, sparkling drinks and in teas. Some extracts are used in cosmetics.

A large number of PS supplements are available.

Active ingredients in American ginseng are panaxosides (saponin glycosides).

Active ingredients in Asian ginseng are ginsenosides (triterpenoid glycosides).

Ginseng products vary considerably in quality because many contain little or no detectable active ingredient.

In few cases, some ginseng products from Asia are mixed with mandrake root, which has been used to induce vomiting, with phenylbutazone or aminopyrine.

The forked root and leaves were traditionally used for medicinal purposes by native Americans.

Since the 18th century, the roots have been collected by "*sang* hunters" and sold to Chinese or traders, who often pay high prices for particularly old wild roots.

Claims: Ginsenosides, unique compounds of the Panax species, are still under intensive, basic and clinical research.

Siberian ginseng, used daily, may increase the number of white blood cells and the activity of the T cells as well as the cytotoxic T cells and natural killer cells that eliminate invading cells and those that have been virally infected.

A study has shown that in patients with herpes simplex virus 2 (which can lead to genital herpes) there was a reduction (of 50%) in the number of outbreaks.

The outbreaks that occurred were less severe and did not last as long.

Ginseng contains significant levels of phytoestrogens. This problem has not been sufficiently evaluated.

Red ginseng (hóng shēn), *P. ginseng*, is a preparation of Gingeng that has been peeled, heated by steaming at boiling temperatures (100°C; 212°F) and then dried (or sun-dried). Red ginseng is frequently marinated in a herbal brew. The resulting roots become extremely brittle.

Ginseng PS extracts and supplements are commonly used according to legendary popular, historical beliefs to enhance physical (including sexual) and mental performance. Ginseng is said to have adaptogenic effects (may increase energy and resistance in contrast to the effects of stress and aging).

Other clinical claims, based on several studies, include reduction of plasma glucose levels, increases in high-density lipoproteins (HDL), hemoglobin and protein levels.

The report of a significant stimulation of the immune system with a possible anticancer effect borders either legend or science fiction (at the moment).

Cardiotonic, endocrine, CNS and estrogenic effects are possibly weak and possibly of an extremely limited clinical value.

Studies have shown that Asian ginseng lowers glucose with possible beneficial effects on immunity.

So far, there is no clear evidence for other significant health claims.

A recent study indicates that a polysaccharide extract of *P. quinquefolius* may be useful in helping prevention of cold episodes and in improving signs and symptoms of subjects with Bechet's disease.

Gummy caramels, used 3–4 times/daily, improve salivation and the level of lysozyme is increased for several hours. This may be effective in reducing the spread of cold and other oral viruses.

Ginseng has been shown to decrease blood alcohol levels.

Adverse effects: Anxiety, nervousness and excitability may occur (on an individual basis); these effects decrease after a few days of use.

Improvement in concentration may decrease, and plasma glucose may become lower (rarely causing hypoglycemia).

Ginseng has a significant estrogen-like effect; therefore, pregnant women or women who are breastfeeding should not use it; it should also be avoided in children.

Rare reports include other side effects (as asthma attacks, increased BP, palpitations, and, in postmenopausal women, some increased risk of uterine bleeding).

For many people, the taste of ginseng is unusual or unpleasant.

Ginseng supplements (considering the dosage) can interact with anti-hyperglycemic drugs, aspirin, NSAIDs, corticosteroids, digoxin, estrogens, MAOIs and anticoagulants.

Characteristic symptoms of acute overdose of Panax ginseng are associated to bleeding.

Symptoms of milder overdose may include dry mouth and lips, excitation, fidgeting, irritability, tremor, palpitations, blurred vision, headache, insomnia, increased body temperature, increased BP, edema, decreased appetite, dizziness, itching, eczema, early morning diarrhea, bleeding and fatigue. Massive overdose with Panax ginseng may cause symptoms including nausea, vomiting, irritability, restlessness, urinary and bowel incontinence, fever, increase in BP, increased respiration rate, decreased sensitivity and reaction to light, decreased heart rate, cyanotic (blue) facial complexion, red facial complexion, seizures, convulsions and delirium.

The possible applications of Ginseng in medicine have not been fully investigated and it is possible that new significant applications will be found in the next years with improvement in technology, extraction and standardization (see Figure 12).

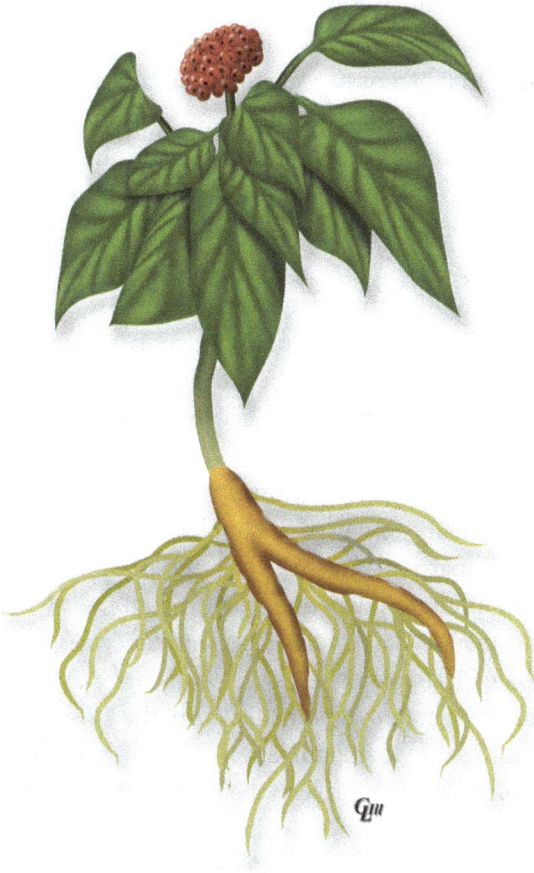

Fig. 12. Ginseng

Glucosamine

In the USA, $C_6H_{13}NO_5$ is one of the most common non-vitamin, non-mineral supplements used by adults.

It is a very well-studied and well-known supplement with several PS products now available.

$C_6H_{13}NO_5$ is an amino sugar precursor in the biochemical synthesis of glycosylated proteins and lipids.

$C_6H_{13}NO_5$ is part of the structure of the polysaccharides-chitosan and chitin the main structural components of exoskeletons of crustaceans and arthropods (also found in the cell walls of fungi and many higher organisms).

$C_6H_{13}NO_5$ is a precursor or multiple cartilage constituents. It is generally extracted from chitin (from the shells of some crabs, from oysters and shrimp); it is used in tablet or capsule form, usually as $C_6H_{13}NO_5$ sulphate, sometimes as $C_6H_{13}NO_5$ hydrochloride.

$C_6H_{13}NO_5$ supplements often include chondroitin sulphate.

Claims: $C_6H_{13}NO_5$ as for other, heavily marketed supplements claims possible benefits on laboratory studies that are of difficult interpretation and clinical meaning.

Some clinical studies are controversial with some trials reporting symptomatic relief from arthritic pain and positive effects on stiffness; some larger studies report minimal benefit in comparison with placebo.

The effects should be considered on the basis of the clinical conditions, presence of inflammation, age, dosages and so many other factors that cannot allow an easy generalization.

There is no evidence to date that supplementation with $C_6H_{13}NO_5$ in athletes and sport participants may prevent or limit joint damage or improve recovery after an injury due to sport trauma.

According to the Merck Manual*, a strong evidence supports the use of $C_6H_{13}NO_5$ sulphate PS supplements in the 'supplementary' management and treatment of mild-moderate symptomatic OA of the knee (usually associated to degeneration and partly to inflammation). Short-term effects tend to affect signs and symptoms and have a role in the treatment of severe knee OA.

A longer supplementation (possibly longer than six months) may positively alter the evolution of osteoarthrosis even modulating the regrowth of cartilage.

The effects of $C_6H_{13}NO_5$ on OA in other anatomical locations (i.e., fingers) or in arthritis and in conditions with a strong inflammatory component (and in younger subjects) are less defined.

Some evidence suggests $C_6H_{13}NO_5$ has both analgesic and anti-inflammatory, disease-modifying effects.

However, evidence from large studies still shows limited and individualized benefit.

One large study indicated that $C_6H_{13}NO_5$ hydrochloride is more beneficial when combined with chondroitin sulphate.

---

*RS Porter and Dr JL Kaplan Ed. The Merck Manual 19 Ed. Merck Sharp & Dohme Corp, Whitehouse st, Nj 2011.

The mechanisms are still not fully clear; clinical improvements may be related to enhanced GAG synthesis due to the sulfate components.

The usual recommended dose is 500 mg *per os* three times a day (tid). With supplementation, $C_6H_{13}NO_5$ concentrations in plasma and synovial fluid increase significantly from baseline levels and the levels in the two fluids are generally highly correlated.

These levels could be biologically advantageous to the articular cartilages if metabolically active.

However, the levels are still 10–100-folds lower than what is theoretically required to improve the cartilage (chondrocytes) and to build new tissue.

$C_6H_{13}NO_5$ sulfate uptake in synovial fluid may be as much as 20%, or could be negligible, indicating minimal biological or clinical significance.

Adverse effects: Allergy has been observed (i.e., in patients who have shellfish allergy); dyspepsia, fatigue, insomnia, headache, some photosensitivity and occasional nail changes may occur.

Concerns about the use in diabetics have been suggested. However, the effects of oral administration of large doses of $C_6H_{13}NO_5$ in animals and the effects of $C_6H_{13}NO_5$ supplementation with normal recommended dosages in humans indicate that $C_6H_{13}NO_5$ does not cause glucose intolerance and has no documented effects on glucose metabolism.

Other studies conducted in lean or obese subjects concluded that oral $C_6H_{13}NO_5$ at standard doses does not cause or significantly worsen insulin resistance or endothelial dysfunction (but these are not clinical parameters and are of dubious clinical value).

There have been some reports of interactions between $C_6H_{13}NO_5$ and other medications; the most significant interaction has been reported with anticoagulants.

FDA and World Health Organization (WHO) medication programs have reported multiple cases with elevated (above safety levels) international normalized ratio (INR) in individuals using anticoagulants (exposing these subjects to a higher risk of bleeding).

Therefore, caution should be used when anticoagulants and $C_6H_{13}NO_5$ are used.

In USA, $C_6H_{13}NO_5$ is not approved by the FDA for medical use.

$C_6H_{13}NO_5$ is classified as a supplement, therefore standards, safety and formulation are the exclusive responsibility of the manufacturer.

Evidence of safety or efficacy is not required as long as it is not advertized or 'claimed' as a treatment for a defined medical condition.

The National Institutes of Health (NIH) is evaluating supplementation with $C_6H_{13}NO_5$ in obese patients since this population may be particularly sensitive to any possible effects of $C_6H_{13}NO_5$ on insulin resistance.

In most of Europe, $C_6H_{13}NO_5$ is approved as a drug and sold in the form of $C_6H_{13}NO_5$ sulfate.

Evidence of safety and efficacy is required for the medical use of $C_6H_{13}NO_5$ as for any other drug and guidelines have recommended its use as an effective and safe therapy for OA.

The use of $C_6H_{13}NO_5$ for some periods (in alternative to other prescription drugs) may reduce the exposure to more 'dangerous' drugs in many patients (i.e., to control phases with a lower degree of symptoms) eventually reducing side effects and chronic complications.

Goldenseal

Goldenseal (*Hydrastis canadensis*) also called orange root or yellow puccoon is considered an an endangered US plant: it is related to the buttercup. In summer, the plant bears a single berry like a large raspberry with 10–30 seeds.

Its active components are hydrastine and berberine, which have antiseptic activity.

Berberine also has shown antidiarrheal properties.

Claims: Goldenseal is used as an antiseptic wash for mouth sores, inflamed and sore eyes, and irritated skin and as a 'soft' cleaning liquid for vaginal infections.

It has been combined with echinacea as a cold remedy, but the efficacy of goldenseal only as a cold remedy has not been proven.

Goldenseal has also been used as a treatment for indigestion and diarrhea.

In two designed studies, berberine, an element isolated from goldenseal, was effective in reducing diarrhea.

Adverse effects: Goldenseal PS supplements may have many adverse effects, including nausea, anxiety, dyspepsia, uterine contractions, jaundice in neonates and it may cause worsening of hypertension.

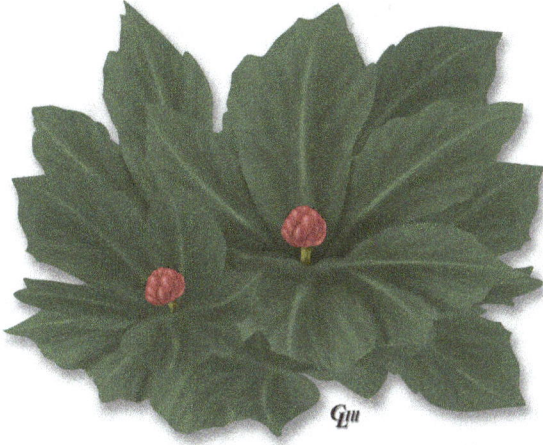

Fig. 13. Goldenseal

If used in large amounts, goldenseal can cause seizures and respiratory failure and may even affect myocardial contraction and cause reduction in left ventricular function.

Goldenseal PS supplements may interact with the anticoagulant warfarin.

Women who are pregnant or breastfeeding, neonates and subjects with a story of seizure disorders or problems with blood clotting should not be treated with goldenseal supplements.

Berberine (a quaternary ammonium salt from the protoberberine group of isoquinoline alkaloids) may reduce the anticoagulant effect of heparin (see Figure 13).

Grape Leaf

Vitis vinifera (common grape vine) is a species of Vitis, native to the Mediterranean region, Central Europe and South Western Asia.

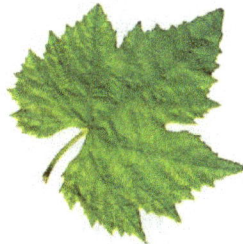

Grape leaf may boost the intake of vitamins being a rich source of the fat-soluble vitamins A and K.

A 1-cup serving of grape leaf contains 3,853 international units of Vitamin A (basically corresponding to one day of recommended intake).

A cup of grape leaf extracts also contains some 15–20 μg of Vitamin K, 17% of the recommended intake for women or 13% for men.

Grape leaf also provides calcium and iron. Medical applications of grape leaf extracts and PS supplements are limited.

Grape leaf extracts are mildly anti-inflammatory compounds.

Chronic inflammation is associated with several conditions (heart disease, many types of cancer, Alzheimer's disease). Other diseases that are associated to inflammation include arthritis and many GI diseases, such as Crohn's disease.

Grape leaves are full of nutrients and have a low glycemic index. According to a study conducted (by the Dermatology at the University of Freiburg), a grape leaf PS supplement may control edema and some symptoms in patients with CVI.

Other uses: Grape leaf — particularly red grape leaves — have been used in the treatment of diarrhea, menstrual bleeding, uterine hemorrhage, some sores and excess vaginal discharge.

Native Americans made grape leaf into a tea for diarrhea, hepatitis, stomachaches and pains.

Grape leaf has a history of being used for a wide variety of conditions, but more research is needed to determine true efficacy.

Grape Seed

Extracts and PS supplements derivate from whole grape seeds with a high concentration of Vitamin E, flavonoids, linoleic acid and phenolic procyanidins (known as oligomeric procyanidins or OPC).

The typical commercial opportunity of extracting grape seed constituents has been known as polyphenols for chemicals having antioxidant activity.

The plant has been selected to produce mainly seeds (dry grape) without a fleshy, watery component. The extracts are produced by carefully selected elements that are, basically, just seed and skin. The production is particularly advanced in grape selection and technology in the Loire Valley.

An important polyphenol contained in grape seeds is resveratrol, which is under evaluation (actually it has been for years) for its possible cardiovascular, antiaging and anticancer effects, an eternal promise.

Other preliminary research on disease models includes management of skin ulcers and wounds as OPCs induce the production of vascular endothelial growth factor and accelerated healing.

In bone physiology, grape seed extracts and PS supplements appear to enhance density and strength (but most work is in animal studies).

OPC may have antiviral and antibacterial effects.·

A recent study has shown efficacy of a grape seed PS supplement in normalizing BP over a short period of time in borderline hypertensives. Also, lipid profiles are marginally but significantly affected with a decrease in cholesterol and triglycerides.

One study in patients with coronary disease and cardiac risk factors found that four weeks of grape seed supplementation caused a minimal improvement in endothelial function (for what it may mean from a clinical point of view).

A meta-analysis of grape seed supplementation confirms that grape seed significantly lowers systolic BP and decreases heart rate with minimal effects on lipids. The study included different patients with different supplements and has a limited clinical meaning. Possibly some subjects respond better to grape seed extracts than others. Again, the suggestion is to try the product for a few weeks (also controlling other risk factors and NaCl intake).

Adverse effects are really uncommon if any. Grape seed PS supplements are used in capsules or tablets usually containing 50 mg or 100 mg. Because of the possible action of proanthocyanidins on decreasing platelet adhesion (in theory), grape seed supplement may theoretically act on coagulation, increasing clotting time.

Grape seed supplements are also an aromatase inhibitor and may suppress the conversion of testosterone to estradiol, but this effect may require really high doses (see Figure 14).

Green Tea

Green tea is made from the leaves from *Camellia sinensis* that have undergone minimal oxidation during processing. Green tea was first brewed in 2737 BC during the reign of Emperor Shennong.

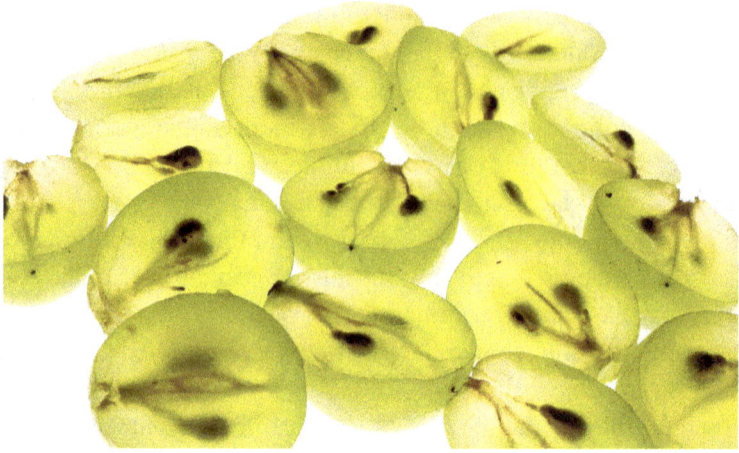

Fig. 14.   Grape

Green tea originated in China, but it has become associated with many cultures throughout Asia. Green tea is made from the leaves of the same plant as traditional tea, an evergreen shrub. The leaves have undergone minimal oxidation during processing.

Traditional tea leaves are fermented, and green tea leaves are steamed but unfermented.

Green tea may be brewed and drunk or ingested in extracted tablet or capsule form in PS supplements.

Green tea supplements have multiple components that are thought to have an important antioxidant and theoretically, anticancer effects.

The supplements of green tea contains polyphenols and catechins as well as caffeine, but many available PS extracts have been decaffeinated.

Green tea also contains a variety of enzymes, amino acids, carbohydrates, lipids, sterols, related compounds, phytochemicals and dietary minerals.

The many claims that have been made for the health benefits of green tea are based on its chemical composition and defined both in *in vitro* and in human studies.

Consuming large (nobody knows how large is large) volumes of green tea and particularly of green tea extracts may lead to oxidative stress and liver toxicity.

As for any anticancer claimed activity, there is no evidence that green tea helps to prevent or treat cancer.

Claims: Green tea is said to have multiple health benefits, none of which are supported by scientific evidence.

As indicated, it has been used for cancer prevention to increase weight loss, to reduce serum lipid reduction, for the prevention of coronary artery disease, for memory enhancement, for the symptomatic relief of OA and pain. Green tea has also been used for the treatment of menopausal symptoms and (for what it means) longevity.

A recent study has indicated that a green tea PS supplement helps to effectively control a defined borderline metabolic syndrome in a group of otherwise healthy subjects in a few weeks.

Adverse effects (rare) are mostly related to effects of caffeine (if present in the supplement).

They include insomnia, anxiety, tachycardia and mild tremor.

Pregnant women should avoid excessive caffeine and tea products as well. Green tea may also interfere with the anticancer drug bortezomib (Velcade) and other boronic acid-based proteasome inhibitors.

A book written by Lu Yu in 600–900 AD (Tang Dynasty), "*Tea Classic*," is considered important in green tea history. The *Kissa Yojoki* (*Book of Tea*), written by Zen priest Eisai in 1191, describes how drinking green tea may affect five vital organs as well as the shapes of tea plants, flowers, leaves and how to grow and process tea leaves.

The new PS supplements may give us the option of better evaluating this plant and its extracts in several preventive and clinical applications which were impossible to study with the tea and extracts only (see Figure 15).

Kava

Kava (or *Kava-Kava*) comes from the roots of a shrub (*Piper methysticum*) that grows in the South Pacific.

The name *kava-kava* is from Tongan and Marquesan. Other names for kava include 'awa (Hawaii), *ava* (Samoa), *yaqona* (Fiji) and *sakau* (Pohnpei).' The roots of the plant are used to produce a drink with sedative and anesthetic properties. Kava is consumed throughout the Pacific.

It is ingested as a tea or in capsule form. Active ingredients are thought to be kavalactones.

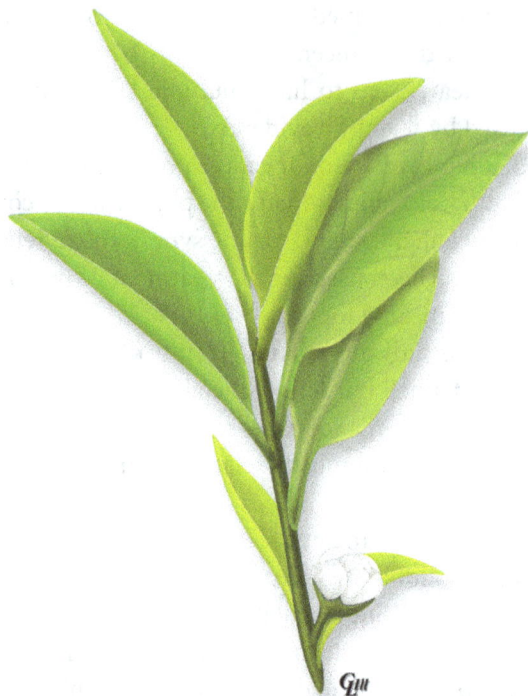

Fig. 15. Green Tea

Kava is a sedating agent and is primarily consumed to relax without disrupting mental clarity.

At least 15 kavalactones have been identified and are all psychoactive. Six of them produce significant effects; their concentrations in kava plants vary.

Different ratios can produce different effects. Supplements include kavalactones extracted from the kava plant using solvents (supercritical carbon dioxide, acetone and ethanol) to produce pills with a standard including between 30% and 90% of kavalactones.

A dose of 150 mg/day of the standardized kava supplements decreases anxiety symptoms.

Most of these studies used a standardized WS 1490 Kava extract formulation, which is composed of 70% kavalactones.

With its unique active ingredients (kavalactones), kava supplements tested in healthy subjects in large studies produced evidence of efficacy in treating short-term social anxiety (whether this is a condition that would need a treatment is open to wild speculations).

People using kava-based supplements have suffered liver damage or liver failure as a result of important levels of hepatotoxicity. Consequently, kava is regulated in a number of countries.

In the EU, it is strictly prohibited in Poland.

Claims: Scientific evidence supports the use of kava as an anxiolytic and sleep aid.

The mechanism is unknown.

Some people use kava for asthma, menopausal symptoms, and UTIs. The dose is 100 mg of standardized extract tid.

Adverse effects: Over 20 people in Europe developed liver toxicity (including liver failure) after taking kava, which induced the FDA to mandate a warning label on kava products. Safety is under continuing surveillance.

When kava is prepared traditionally (as tea) and used in high doses (>6–12 g/day of dried root) or over long periods (up to six weeks), there have been reports of scaly skin rash (kava dermopathy), blood changes (e.g., macrocytosis, leukopenia) and neurologic changes (e.g., torticollis, oculogyric crisis, worsening of Parkinson's disease, movement disorders).

Also, kava may prolong the effect of other sedatives (e.g., barbiturates) and affect driving or other activities requiring alertness.

Heavy kava use in an aboriginal community in Arnhem Land was associated with overall poor health, a puffy face, scaly rash and a slight increase in patellar reflexes.

A 2012 analysis of cases worldwide proposed that mould was the primary cause of hepatotoxicity in kava products.

In 2002, the EU imposed a ban on imports of kava-based pharmaceutical products.

The sale of kava plant is regulated in Switzerland, France and Netherlands. Some Pacific Island States who had been benefiting from the export of kava to the pharmaceutical companies have attempted to overturn the EU ban on kava-based pharmaceutical products by invoking international trade agreements at the WTO: Fiji, Samoa, Tonga and Vanuatu argued that the ban was imposed with insufficient evidence.

The pressure prompted Germany to reconsider the evidence base for banning kava-based pharmaceutical products.

In the United Kingdom, kava is considered a recreational, illegal drug and it is a criminal offence to sell, supply or import any medicinal product containing kava.

Exclusion of certain aerial parts of the plant (when preparing the extract of supplements) is also often required by law or convention. The extract contains less pipermethystine and other toxic compounds.

The use of kava is basically a local tradition in islands with a different (from Western Societies) type of life and customs. In some parts of Australia (Northern Territory), the police considers the sale and, in majority of circumstances, possession of kava 'illegal'.

In most cases, kava is used and marketed just as recreational drugs. It is used for medicinal, religious, political, cultural and social uses throughout the Pacific.

These cultures have a great respect for the plant and place a high importance on it.

In Fiji, a formal *yaqona* (kava) ceremony will often accompany important social, political, religious functions, involving a ritual presentation of the bundled roots as a *sevusevu* (gift).

Some of its effects may have a significant medical value, but this supplement — if it is a supplement — needs important studies.

Licorice

Licorice is derived from the root of *Glycyrrhiza glabra*. The root can also be eaten as it is. A sweet flavor can be extracted from the root. The liquorice plant is a legume that is native to southern Europe, India and parts of Asia. It is not botanically related to anise, star anise, or fennel, which include similar flavoring compounds. Licorice root has been around since ancient times. It was found in great quantities in the tomb of King Tut among gold, jewelry and treasures. It was suggested that King Tut wanted to take the root with him on his journey to the next world. For Egyptians, Licorice root was a cure-all (as ginseng was for the Chinese). The Scythians were able to go 12 days without drinking water because they chewed on Licorice root. It was considered very good for coughs and all respiratory diseases. Around 80 AD, Pliny suggested the use of Licorice to clear the voice and to alleviate thirst and hunger. Dioscorides gave the plant its botanical name (Greek glukos = sweet, riza = root). He traveled with Alexander the Great; he told the soldiers to chew Licorice to stop thirst when water was scarce and to give them stamina and endurance during long marches.

Natural licorice has a very characteristic sweet taste; it has also been used medicinally as capsules, tablets or extracts.

Now, most licorice candies are flavored artificially and do not contain natural licorice. Glycyrrhizin is the active ingredient in natural licorice.

For people sensitive to the effects of glycyrrhizin, products that contain a much lower amount of glycyrrhizin (about one-tenth) are available (deglycyrrhizinated licorice).

Claims: Licorice may help to control or suppress coughs, it may sooth a sore throat and is used to relieve stomach upset.

When applied topically, it used to improve skin irritation and eczema.

There are not enough studies to define whether licorice is effective for improving stomach ulcers or gastitis, or complications associated to hepatitis C.

This supplement has been proposed as being useful for liver protection in tuberculosis therapy, but there is no clear evidence.

Liquorice and PS supplements may be effective in controlling hyperlipidaemia and some studies showed some efficacy in treating inflammation-induced skin pigmentation.

Liquorice may also be effective in preventing some neurodegenerative disorders and even dental caries.

The laxative, antidiabetic, anti-inflammatory, immunomodulatory and anti-tumoral activities are under evaluation.

The expectorant properties of liquorice are well-known and have also been under investigation with conflicting results.

Liquorice is very popular in Italy (particularly in the South) and in Spain in its natural form or as black soft or hard candies and gummies.

The root of the plant is simply dug up, cleaned, washed and chewed. Throughout Italy, unsweetened liquorice is consumed in the form of small black pieces made only from 100% pure liquorice extract; the taste is bitter, intense and very typical.

In these forms, it is not a supplement but just a candy.

Adverse effects: High doses of licorice and glycyrrhizin may cause renal Na and water retention even leading to higher BP and potassium excretion.

This may cause low potassium levels. Increased potassium excretion can pose problem for patients with heart disease if they use digoxin or diuretics that also increase potassium excretion. These patients should avoid licorice.

Licorice may increase the risk of premature delivery; theoretically, pregnant women should avoid licorice.

The isoflavene glabrene and the isoflavane glabridin, found in the roots of liquorice, are considered phytoaestrogens (see Figure 16).

Mangosteen

Purple mangosteen (*Garcinia mangostana*), known as **mangosteen**, is a tropical evergreen tree believed to have originated in the Sunda Islands and the Moluccas of Indonesia.

Mangosteen peel contains xanthonoids, such as mangostin and other phytochemicals having antioxidant properties.

Some studies demonstrated that juice containing mangosteen peel extracts may reduce blood levels of C-reactive protein, a biomarker of inflammation.

Research on the phytochemistry of the plant without human clinical study is inadequate to assure the real safety or efficacy of its use as a supplement. No side effects have been reported.

Some mangosteen juice products contain whole fruit purée or polyphenols extracted from the inedible exocarp (rind). The resulting juice has purple color and astringency derived from exocarp pigments.

Different parts of the plant have a significant history of use in medicine, mainly in Southeast Asia.

It has been used to treat skin infections, difficult wounds, dysentery and UTIs, but studies are very limited at the moment.

Melatonin

The jet-setter status symbol is also a hormone produced by the pineal gland. It helps in regulating circadian rhythm and sleep. It is derived from animal's

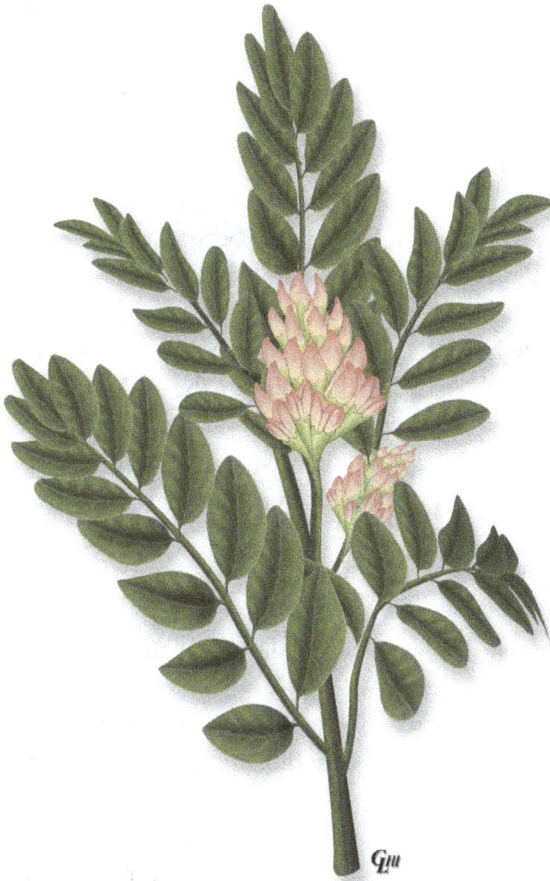

Fig. 16. Licorice

sources, but it can be also produced synthetically. In some countries, melatonin is considered a drug and is regulated as such; **5-methoxytryptamine** is a hormone found in animals, plants, fungi and bacteria. It is the most fundamental and universal hormone in the evolution of cellular life, primarily acting as an antioxidant against the Sun's radiation.

It is synthesized in animal cells directly from the aminoacid tryptophan, but in other organisms through the Shikimic acid pathway, in response to dark-light period alternance.

Melatonin is categorized by the FDA as a supplement. There are several PS supplements.

It is sold over-the-counter in US and Canada without any regulation as a pharmaceutical drug. FDA regulations applying to medications are not applicable to melatonin. However, FDA rules required that by June 2010, all production of dietary supplements must comply with "current good manufacturing practices" (cGMP) and be manufactured with "controls that result in a consistent product free of contamination with accurate labelling."

The industry has also been required to report to the FDA all serious adverse events, and the FDA has (within the cGMP guidelines) begun enforcement of that requirement.

Claims: Some scientific evidence suggests use of melatonin to minimize the effects of jet lag, especially in people travelling eastward over two to five time zones. In one large study, melatonin supplements did not relieve symptoms of jet lag. However, jet lag is not easy to evaluate and it is not a disease.

At the moment, only a few small studies suggest that these supplements can be used to treat insomnia.

Melatonin can be taken orally as capsules, tablet or liquid. It is also available in a form to be used sublingually and there are transdermal patches.

Standard dosage is not established and ranges from 0.5 to 5 mg taken 1 h before usual bedtime on the day of travel and two to four nights after arrival.

The evidence supporting use of melatonin as a sleep aid in adults and children with neuropsychiatric disorders (e.g., pervasive developmental disorders) is quite weak.

Melatonin has also been studied as a potential treatment of gastro-esophageal reflux, some immune disorders, depression, seasonal affective disorder (SAD) (if this is a medical entity), circadian rhythm sleep disorders and even sexual dysfunction and insomnia in the elderly. However, in most studies, limited results were observed.

Melatonin can alter electrophysiological processes associated with memory, such as long-term potentiation (LTP).

Melatonin has been tested in Alzheimer's disease. Supplementation with melatonin is considered a possible, effective preventive treatment for migraines and cluster headaches.

Adverse effects are hangover, drowsiness, headache and transient depression that may occur in some subjects.

Melatonin may worsen cases of depression. Theoretically, prion infection caused by products derived from neurologic tissues of some animals could be a risk.

Melatonin can lower follicle-stimulating hormone (FSH) levels.

Effects of the hormone on human reproduction remain unclear, although it was tried (with some effects) as a contraceptive in the 1990s.

Symptoms of Parkinson's disease may be affected. Both hyperthyroidism and hypothyroidism may be affected. Melatonin protects against cell damage, but it may also down-regulate the activity of the thyroid gland.

In some cases, melatonin could worsen hypothyroidism.

Subjects using melatonin should avoid activities that require alertness — i.e., driving or operating heavy machinery — for 4–5 h after taking melatonin.

Melatonin is generally recommended only for short-term use (about two months).

Milk Thistle

Milk Thistle (MT) is a purple-flowered plant. *Silybum marianum* has other common names (**cardus marianus, MT, blessed MT, Marian thistle, Mary Thistle, Saint Mary's thistle, Mediterranean MT, variegated thistle** and **Scotch thistle**).

This species is an annual or biennial plant of the Asteraceae family. Its sap and seeds contain the active ingredient silymarin, a potent antioxidant and hepatothropic agent.

The extracts include some 65–80% silymarin (a flavonolignan complex) and 20–35% fatty acids including linoleic acid.

Silymarin is a complex mixture of polyphenolic molecules, including seven closely related flavonolignans (silybin A, silybin B, isosilybin A, isosilybin B, silychristin, isosilychristin, silydianin) and one major flavonoid (taxifolin).

Silibinin, a semipurified fraction of silymarin, is primarily a mixture of two diastereoisomers, silybin A and silybin B, in an approximate 1:1 ratio.

Silibinin (sylimarin I) appears to have many significant hepatoprotective, hepatothrophic activities and anti-hepatotoxic activities that may protect liver cells against some toxins.

In vitro research has indicated that silibinin is clearly hepato protective. MT extracts and PS supplements both prevent and repair damage to the liver from toluene and/or xylene.

Workers exposed to toxic vapors from toluene or xylene for years used a PS MT supplement with 80% silymarin for 30 days. The workers using the supplement showed significant improvement in liver function tests [alanine transaminase (ALT) and aspartate transaminase (AST)] and platelet counts.

A study in 2010 found that eight major compounds in silybum, including seven flavonolignans — silybin A, silybin B, isosilybin A, isosilybin B, silychristin, isosilychristin, silydianin and one flavonoid, taxifolin — are inhibitors of hepatitis C virus (HCV) ribonucleic acid (RNA)-dependent RNA polymerase, suggesting a significant potential in specifically treating liver damage linked to HCV.

Silymarin supplementation (140 mg orally three times daily) appears to have some but limited effects when used for one year in combination with ursodeoxycholic acid (UDCA) in the management of primary biliary cirrhosis.

MT supplementation was associated with a trend towards reducing some liver damaging effects of chemotherapy in a study involving 50 children.

In clinical studies, silymarin has typically been used in oral doses ranging from 420 to 480 mg/day (in two to three divided doses). Higher doses have been evaluated (600 mg daily in the treatment of patients with type II diabetes and 600–1200 mg daily in patients with chronic HCV).

Optimization of dosage, solubility and administration plans have not been defined or standardized.

MT (with dandelion and other extracts) have been considered hangover cures as the bitter tincture may help organs to eliminate alcohol after heavy drinking.

Claims: MT is said to treat cirrhosis (or control its evolution) and to protect the liver from viral hepatitis. Also, it may attenuate the damaging effects of alcohol and protect liver from the effects of some hepatotoxic drugs.

In *in vitro* studies, silymarin increases the levels of intrahepatic glutathione, an antioxidant considered important for detoxification.

Studies have been unable to show that MT PS supplements offer a significant benefit to people with severe liver disease.

However, the studies should focus on very specific conditions as the causes of liver damage can be diverse, and very often there is more than one cause. There is no way to improve functions in dead cells without a metabolic value.

There are individual case reports that claim fatality reduction in acute mushroom poisoning.

Results indicate that severe liver damage due to *Amanita phalloides* liver cell necrosis can be prevented effectively when administration of silybin begins within 48 h of mushroom intake. Other case control studies also suggest that silibinin reduces mortality from mushroom poisoning.

Other uses to be clinically verified indicate that MT supplementation may lower cholesterol levels and reduce cell damage caused by radiation (and chemotherapy), reduce insulin resistance in people with type 2 diabetes with cirrhosis. There is some indication that MT supplements may reduce the growth of some cancer cells (breast, cervical, prostate cancers) and even have some effects in patients with Alzheimer's disease (both in prevention and treatment). At the moment, there is no way to translate this information into clinically useful treatments.

Studies and results are very limited and these problems are very complex.

A recent Indian multicentre study on more than 650 patients in different levels and conditions associated with liver damage indicated that a new PS supplement (liverubin) is generally effective in decreasing liver damage (considering enzymes) in weeks without any side effect. Another study in moderate, temporary liver damage also has shown the efficacy of the same supplement.

A potential favourable action of PS supplements could be considered when giving patients drugs or treatments that may potentially cause liver damage or when patients are at higher risk of liver damage.

Adverse effects: No significant adverse effects have been reported with MT. New PS supplements are now produced with improved absorption and efficacy.

MT may increase the effects of antihyperglycemic drugs and may theoretically interfere with indinavir.

Women with hormone-sensitive conditions (breast, uterine and ovarian cancers; endometriosis; uterine fibroids) should theoretically avoid MT supplements.

Sylimarin can be considered a *'cell protector'*.

Studies on kidney protection and on the protection of other organs (including the arterial wall) are in progress.

A human study in prostate cancer (aimed to study the effects of high dose of silibinin) observed that 13 g daily are well tolerated in patients with advanced prostate cancer.

The compound does not have embryotoxic potential (in animal models) (see Figure 17).

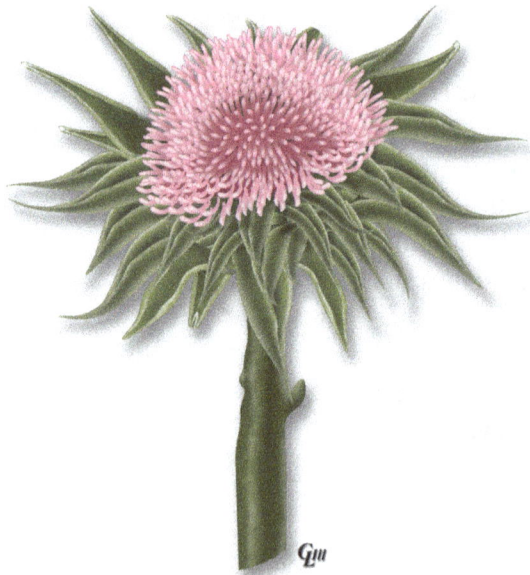

Fig. 17. Milk Thistle

Nattokinase

Nattokinase (NKCP) is a purified filtrate of *bacillus subtilis* natto culture.

Natto is a traditional Japanese food made with fermented soybeans. The *Bacillus subtilis* natto (formed in the fermentation process) produces functional proteins (including NKCP) which maintain optimum blood viscosity and thrombogenicity.

NKCP helps reducing the risk of thrombosis possibly in both the arterial and venous circulation.

Deep vein thrombosis (DVT) occurring during or after long flights may be partially prevented by NKCP.

Natto as a food may contain large amounts of Vitamin K2 which may interfere with warfarin. **NKCP** (nattokinase, Daiwa) is a specific PS supplement of natto bacillus culture (Bacillopeptidase F) used (tablets 125 mg) for preventing thrombotic conditions.

Several enzymes have been identified in NKCP, including NKCP. These enzymes inactivate in the blood plasminogen activator inhibitor (PAI-1) which tends to increase with age. By reducing PAI-1, NKCP increases the efficiency of blood control mechanisms associated with viscosity. NKCP does not directly act upon blood viscosity and does not dissolve blood clots.

The supplemement increases the efficiency of blood control mechanisms including spontaneous fibrinolysis. Therefore, NKCP does not alter normal blood coagulation or platelet aggregation.

Safety: NKCP safety has been evaluated in clinical studies. No clinical adverse effects were seen with dosages between 750 mg/day and 1250 mg/day.

A dose of 250–500 mg of NKCP (2–4 tablets) is recommended as the standard dose per day (after the evening meal).

NKCP has a thrombolytic effect *in vitro* and *in vivo* after ingestion. The effect is milder when compared to the plasminogen activator (t-PA). NKCP has been confirmed to decompose and inactivate PAI-1 in cell culture systems. Oral NKCP administration for days reduces the PAI-1 and helps the t-PA to work more efficiently; t-PA activates plasmin and reduces blood fibrin. Therefore, NKCP facilitates the activation of the spontaneous fibrinolysis cascade by reducing PAI-1 and maintains the balance between coagulation and fibrinolysis. NKCP ingestion is unlikely to dissolve fibrin excessively causing clinical problems (i.e., bleeding).

NKCP ingestion is unlikely to cause unexpected fibrinolysis.

NKCP has been used to prevent thrombosis in long flights (in a association with Pycnogenol in a specific combination define a Flite Tabs). NKCP has been also used to prevent recurrent DVT after an epidode of major DVT and for the prevention of new episodes of retinal thrombosis.

However, data (on file) are not widely available.

Pycnogenol

In his Berlin laboratories, Charles Haimoff developed a unique substance, a water-soluble flavonoid extract from the bark of the French maritime pine tree, called Pycnogenol.

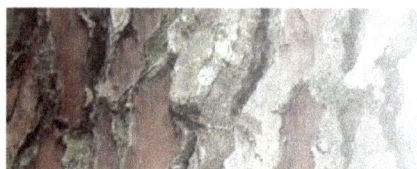

Pycnogenol extract (unique, PS standardized supplement) is a potent blend of antioxidants, a natural anti-inflammatory agent.

The product stimulates the generation of collagen and hyaluronic acid and improves the natural vasomotor activity of blood vessels by supporting production of nitric oxide.

It is one of the most studied (3rd generation) supplements and it is considered a case model for all PS supplements development, standardization and evaluation.

Pycnogenol® helps in maintaining a physiological microcirculation by improving the relaxation of arteries, when needed, according to physiological needs.

Consequently, Pycnogenol improves perfusion in many organs and modulates BP.

The antioxidant activity of Pycnogenol protects the skin from the free radicals produced by ultraviolet (UV) exposure and environmental damage.

Pycnogenol has been tested in several arthrosis studies as a supplementary treatment. It improves joint mobility and flexibility and its anti-inflammatory activity helps in relieving signs/symptoms associated with both degenerative and inflammatory arthrosis.

Pycnogenol has also been used to improve retinal circulation — reducing edema — in diabetics with microangiopathy.

Supplementation with Pycnogenol controls some cardiovascular risk factors with improvement in BP in borderline hypertensive subjects and by modulating platelet adhesion.

Also, blood lipids and blood sugar values may be improved in most cardiovascular subjects with a positive interaction with 'standard' treatments and risk-control management.

Several studies show — in different type of studies — the effects of Pycnogenol supplementation in controlling the most significant cardiovascular risk factors.

Circulation studies have found that this supplement increases the induced vasodilation of arteries (when altered) in cardiovascular patients.

BP studies in hypertensives have shown that Pycnogenol improves the physiological vasodilatory response after reactive hyperemia.

It has a positive interaction with other drugs used to control risk factors.

With Pycnogenol, cholesterol may be reduced in selected cardiovascular patients and in most subjects at risk. Supplementation with Pycnogenol tends to increases high-density lipoprotein (HDL) cholesterol.

The supplement has also shown an important activity in subjects with arthrosis by improving symptoms in association with lowering inflammatory markers (including C-reative protein) and oxidative stress.

In these patients, Pycnogenol limits the activation of the pro-inflammatory protein complex NF-κB.

As a consequence, subjects treated with this PS supplement generate less matrix metalloproteinase (MMP)

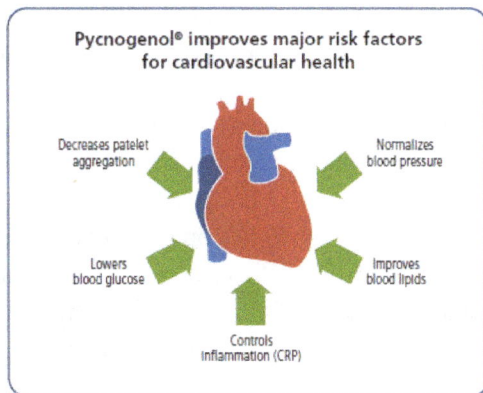

Pycnogenol® improves major risk factors for cardiovascular health

Decreases patelet aggregation

Normalizes blood pressure

Lowers blood glucose

Improves blood lipids

Controls Inflammation (CRP)

enzymes (responsible for the degeneration of cartilage collagen in OA). The supplement also inhibits the generation of COX-2 enzymes in inflammation, lowering pain.

In sports, Pycnogenol has shown efficacy in improving physical performance; athletes showed an increase of endurance with the supplement. In one study, the athletes performed under controlled conditions (on a treadmill). The study showed a significant increase of endurance with Pycnogenol.

The supplement improves muscle recovery and muscular pain associated to fatigue and alleviates the occurrence of cramps.

In venous disease (uncomplicated varicose veins) and in CVI, Pycnogenol improves edema — the hallmark of CVI — that may progress to more serious complications (including ulcerations) if left untreated.

At least 15 clinical studies have been published on venous insufficiency and CVI.

In this field, Pycnogenol has a very strong documentation. The higher efficacy of Pycnogenol as a venous insufficiency management and treatment tool (in comparison with other products) is obvious in several studies. Pycnogenol is more effective than horse chestnut extracts, but it is also comparatively more effective than any other treatment for CVI with a power factor of 10 (a dose some 10 times higher is needed for other products to have some effects, comparable to the effects produced by Pycnogenol).

Pycnogenol produces more significant results on CVI symptoms than other products.

This supplement also reduces edema due to long flights. Long periods of immobility, a dry atmosphere and small airplane cabin space are contributing factors to leg swelling due to limited venous circulation; fluids tend to accumulate in distal tissues. Leg and ankle swelling are also associated to vein thrombosis.

In recent studies on flight-related swelling, it was found that Pycnogenol has a positive effect on leg swelling and edema during long flights (lasting 7–12 hours).

More recent studies on cognitive functions and an acute model study on jet lag associated to some cognitive impairment indicate an improvement in cognitive functions in healthy individuals.

This observation may be physiologically related to the control of water (and edema) within the cerebral tissue.

Tinnitus and Meniere's syndrome have been improved in more limited studies by supplementation with Pycnogenol.

Two other studies have indicated that Pycnogenol supplementation may reduce the course of common cold of at least one day and reduce the incidence of tracheal and pulmonary complications.

Studies on asthma and psoriasis have shown very interesting results.

The product behaves as a general, natural anti-inflammatory agent and effectively controls the genesis and evolution of edema (including subclinical edema) associated to several clinical conditions.

Many applications with different dosages (30–200 mg/day) have been made available.

Microcirculation has also been selectively evaluated in several studies that have indicated its efficacy (i.e., in diabetic microangiopathy and vasospastic conditions).

Important, recent studies have indicated that Pycnogenol may slow down the progression of atherosclerotic plaques in selected individuals and the progression from asymptomatic to symptomatic cardiovascular stages in subjects with more significant, stenotic plaques.

The atherosclerosis study is still in progress and it is very promising.

This study uses a combination of Pycnogenol and a specific *Centella Asiatica* PS supplement.

Pycnogenol is now available also in thin skin patches. Initial results indicate an important anti-inflammatory action and a decrease in oxidative stress after patch application.

Adverse effects: No clinically significant adverse effect has been observed.

The product is very safe and well tolerated and so far, no significant adverse interactions with other treatments or drugs have been observed (see Figure 18).

Quercetin

Quercetin is a flavonol complex found in many fruits, vegetables, leaves and grains. The name is derived from Quercus.

It is a naturally occurring polar auxin transport inhibitor. Quercetin is present in various kinds of honey from different plant sources.

The enzyme quercitrinase can be found in *Aspergillus flavus*. Its substrates are quercitrin and H_2O that releases quercetin and L-rhamnose. It is

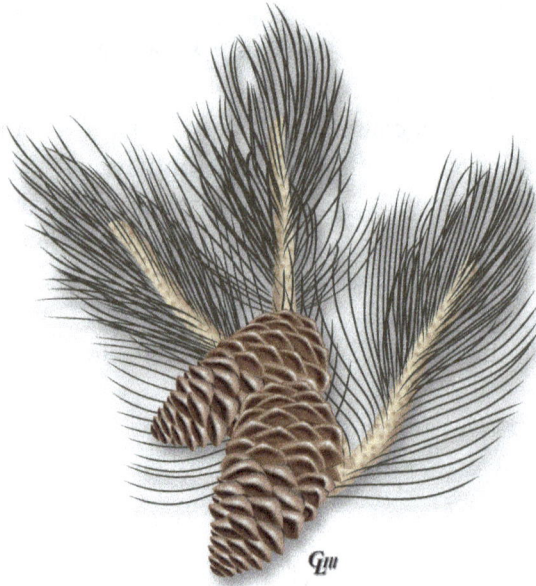

Fig. 18. Pinus Pinaster bark is used to produce Pycnogenol

an enzyme in the rutin catabolic pathway. Quercetin 3-O-sulfate is a human plasma quercetin metabolite.

Quercetin is the aglycone form of a number of other flavonoid glycosides, such as rutin and quercitrin, found in citrus fruit, buckwheat and onions. Quercetin forms the glycosides quercitrin and rutin together with rhamnose and rutinose, respectively.

CTN-986 is a quercetin derivative found in cottonseeds and cotton-seed oil. Miquelianin is the quercetin 3-O-β-D-glucopyranoside.

Quercetin may induce insulin secretion by activation of L-type calcium channels in pancreatic β-cells.

Quercetin is used for empirically treating conditions of the heart including atherosclerosis, high cholesterol and to control cardiovascular risk factors.

PS supplements based on quercetin are also used in subjects with diabetes, cataracts, hay fever, peptic ulcer, schizophrenia (no real indications or evidence), inflammatory conditions, asthma, gout, viral infections and in benign prostatic hyperthrophy.

Quercetin PS supplements are also used to increase endurance and improve athletic performance with very limited evidence.

Supplements of quercetin have antioxidant and anti-inflammatory effects that need to be evaluated using PS products.

Currently, there is no defined clinical or preventive application.

The FDA has issued warning letters to emphasize that quercetin is not a defined nutrient, cannot be assigned a dietary content level and is not regulated as a drug to treat any human disease.

Adverse effects: Quercetin is contraindicated with some antibiotics. It may interact with fluoroquinolones (quercetin competitively binds to bacterial DNA gyrase).

Whether this inhibits or enhances the effect of fluoroquinolones is not clear.

The American Hospital Formulary Service (AHFS) Drug Information specifically names quercetin as a compound with potential harmful interactions with taxol.

As paclitaxel is metabolized primarily by CYP2C8, its bioavailability may be increased unpredictably, potentially leading to harmful side effects.

Robuvit

Robuvit is a new, highly standardized, PS supplement produced from a wood extract from *quercus robur* (French oak). Robuvit includes several ellagitannins that have major antioxidant and anti-inflammatory actions with an important effect on distal edema (i.e., in lymphatic patients).

Human absorption of specific roburins from a French oak wood extract (Robuvit) can be measured by evaluating the plasmatic increase of total phenols and the appearance of some roburin metabolites.

Supplementation with Robuvit increases the global plasma antioxidant capacity.

Cell cultures have assessed the action of metabolites on gene expression modulation in endothelial, neuronal, and keratinocyte cell lines. Robuvit metabolites appear to affect ribosome, cell cycle and spliceosome pathways.

However, these cellular effects are difficult to compare to actual human, clinical models.

Robuvit extract concentrates water-soluble components of the wood (defined as ellagitannins) also found in wine that has been resting in oak barrels for years. Flavors are imported into the wine from the wood as it ages in oak barrels. The use of oak has been prevalent in winemaking for centuries. These substances derived from oak wood are considered completely safe. Wine in the barrel acquires different types of tannins.

The specific PS supplement from oak wood is specified to contain in its composition at least 20% of roburins (A, B, C, D and E) and grandinin. Both components belong to the group of hydrolysable tannins (also defined ellagitannins).

Clinical investigations in healthy volunteers and patients in different clinical conditions have preliminarily shown an increased antioxidant capacity of the blood after supplementation.

Also, a significant decrease in peripheral edema after supplementation with Robuvit has been observed.

Lymphatic edema (mainly primary lymphedema and lymphedema secondary to surgery or radiotherapy) is specifically affected.

The most important hydrolysable tannins included in Robuvit may be effective — the supplement is under evaluation — in different preclinical and clinical conditions (associated with chronic inflammation) as they have a basic anti-inflammatory action.

The product is active at a dosage between 100 and 300 mg. The strong antioxidant efficacy of Robuvit has been tested in healthy volunteers (improving oxidative stress), in patients with hepatic failure with good results on hepatic functional values.

Data from this pilot, supplement registry study indicate a significant protective activity of Robuvit, associated with a very good safety profile, in patients with temporary hepatic failure. The activity of Robuvit® seems to be mediated by its combined antioxidant and anti-inflammatory activity.

Robuvit has also been effective in the management of subjects with chronic fatigue syndrome and increased oxidative stress. These subjects improved with Robuvit supplementation in comparison with untreated controls.

No side effects have been observed during or after Robuvit supplementation so far.

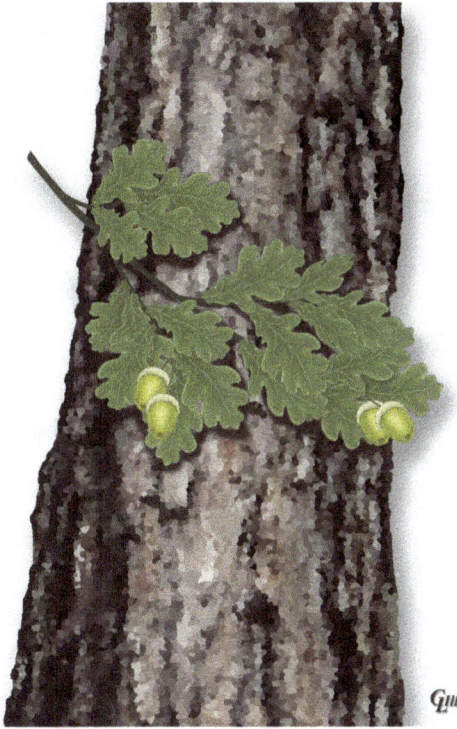

Fig. 19. Robuvit

Robuvit is still in development and it could be considered the first PS supplement of this kind (see Figure 19).

S-Adenosyl-L-Methionine

S-Adenosyl-L-Methionine (SAM) is a derivative of methionine and a cofactor for multiple synthetic pathways. It is produced naturally in the body and manufactured synthetically in several PS supplement forms.

It is a common cosubstrate involved in methyl group transfers.

SAM was discovered in Italy by GL Cantoni in 1952. It is produced from ATP and by methionine adenosyltransferase. Transmethylation, trans-sulfuration, and aminopropylation are the metabolic pathways that use SAM. These anabolic reactions occur anywhere in the body, but most SAM is produced and consumed in the liver.

The product is a Standard Process (SP) supplement or a drug in some countries.

Claims: SAM is said to be effective for treatment of depression, OA and liver disorders, but scientific studies, so far, are limited and do not confirm these claims.

More research is needed to verify its clinical efficacy.

Some research, including clinical trials, where the product is considered a drug, and specific claims should indicate that SAM, used on a regular basis, may help in the management of depression.

SAM may have some positive effects in the treatment of functional liver diseases and may help in the chronic management of pain and inflammation in patients with symptomatic OA, helping to control symptoms.

The Dietary Supplement Health and Education Act (1994) allows the distribution of SAM as a supplement by passing the regulatory requirements for drugs (by the FDA).

When a series of studies found evidence of abnormally low levels of endogenous SAM (that, theoretically, may have a role in the evolution of Alzheimer's disease), SAM was considered to have therapeutic potential in this field.

However, further research has indicated this effect is likely due to Vitamin B_{12} deficiencies, which cause some of the neurological alterations (due to the inability to conduct one carbon transfers with folate in the absence of Vitamin B_{12}).

Very low levels of SAM have been found in the cerebrospinal fluid and in other brain regions in Alzheimer's disease patients.

However, this clinical line of research is almost impossible to define and to follow due to costs, prolonged times and variability of clinical patterns.

Small studies have not shown a consistent effect of SAM on homocysteine levels.

High levels of homocysteine may be associated with atherosclerosis and an increased risk of heart attacks, strokes, liver damage, and possibly Alzheimer's disease. Vitamin B supplements are often used and taken with SAM. These vitamins help metabolize homocysteine into other compounds controlling increased levels.

Adverse effects: No serious adverse effects have been reported. SAM is contraindicated in patients with bipolar disorder because SAM can precipitate manic episodes. GI disorder, dyspepsia and anxiety can occur with SAM supplements.

Long-term effects are for the most part unknown.

SAM is a weak DNA-alkylating agent.

When used with some drugs this may increase the risk of serotonin syndrome, a potentially dangerous condition caused by having too much serotonin.

These drugs include dextromethorphan (Robitussin), meperidine (Demerol), pentazocine (Talwin) and tramadol (Ultram).

SAM may also interact with some antidepressant medications increasing the potential for their side effects and reduce the effectiveness of levodopa for Parkinson's disease.

Saw Palmetto

The Mayans drank SP as a tonic and the Seminoles used the berries as an expectorant and antiseptic.

The extract of SP is produced from the fruit of *Serenoa repens* rich in fatty acids and phytosterols. PS supplements have been used to treat a variety of conditions, mostly benign prostatic hyperplasia (BPH).

Recent clinical trials found the extract to be more effective than placebo for BPH. However, the Merck Manual clearly indicates SP as an effective supplement for BPH.

Only berries from SP contain the plant's active ingredients in reasonable quantities. The active ingredients (possibly fatty acids) are still partially unidentified, but they appear to inhibit 3a-reductase opposing the conversion of testosterone to dihydro-testosterone.

Palmetto PS supplements used in recent studies are made with hexane extracts of SP berries including some 80–90% of essential fatty acids and phytosterols.

Claims: Strong scientific evidence supports use of SP PS supplements to treat symptoms of BPH (e.g., frequent urination, dysuria, etc.).

Clinical evidence — not completely documented — suggests that it may reverse at least partially, in time, hyperplasia.

But some large studies did not show any benefit on the evolution of hyperplasia.

There are claims that SP supplements may increase sperm production, breast size, or sexual vigor in younger men, but these results are basically unproven.

For PS supplements, doses are 320 mg once a day or 160 mg bid.

Generally, some two months are needed to detect significant improvements in signs and symptoms in most patients.

At the moment, SP extract and supplements are the most popular 'plant-derived' treatment for BPH.

Patients can try the product and evaluate individual effects and decide whether to continue with supplements or switch to prescription drugs that have some significant side effects.

A PS supplement that combine echinacea and SP has shown to be effective — more than Palmetto alone — in controlling signs/symptoms of BPH.

Adverse effects: Headache and diarrhea in some subjects have been documented.

Beta-sitosterol, a chemical present in SP extract, is chemically similar to cholesterol. High levels of sitosterol concentrations in blood have correlated with increased severity of atherosclerosis and heart disease in men who previously suffered heart attacks.

No other serious adverse effects have been reported so far. The product is considered generally very safe.

SP supplements may theoretically interact with estrogen; thus, women who are pregnant or who may become pregnant should not take it (but the supplement is mainly used by men).

SP extracts can slow down clotting, theoretically leading to increased bleeding before and after surgery.

Patients taking SP may have increased bleeding time during surgery.

The bleeding time returns to normal after the patient stops supplementation.

The use of SP supplements should also be stopped at least two weeks before a scheduled surgical procedure.

Also, effects on the coagulation and aggregation can be seen in association with antiplatelets agents (see Figure 20).

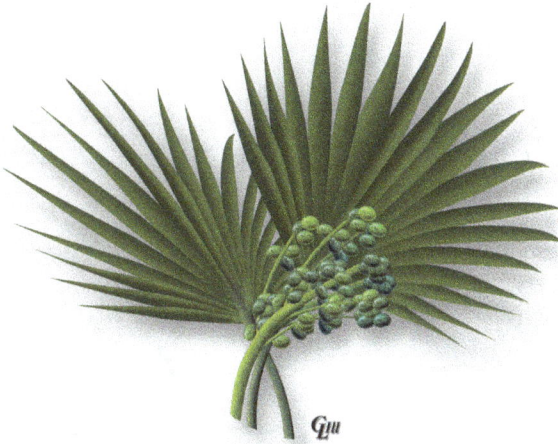

Fig. 20. Saw Palmetto

Sophora Japonica

Sophora japonica is a species of tree in the subfamily Faboideae of the pea family Fabaceae. Theoretically, it has abortifacient, antibacterial, anticholesterolemic, anti-inflammatory, antispasmodic, diuretic, emetic, emollient, febrifuge, hypotensive, purgative, styptic and tonic properties. *S. japonicum* contains the isoflavone glycoside sophoricoside.

The Chinese name for the tree (槐) is composed of the word 木 ("wood") and 鬼 ("demon"). It appears that the presence of this tree keeps away other plants by different poisonus substances.

It has been used in the treatment of CVI and varicose veins in several PS supplements.

It is a major component of a leading venous product (Venoruton-Paroven, Novartis) (see Figure 21).

St. John's Wort

Hypericum perforatum is a flowering plant species of the genus *Hypericum*. It is a medicinal herb with significant antidepressant properties and potential antibacterial and anti-inflammatory properties (arachidonate

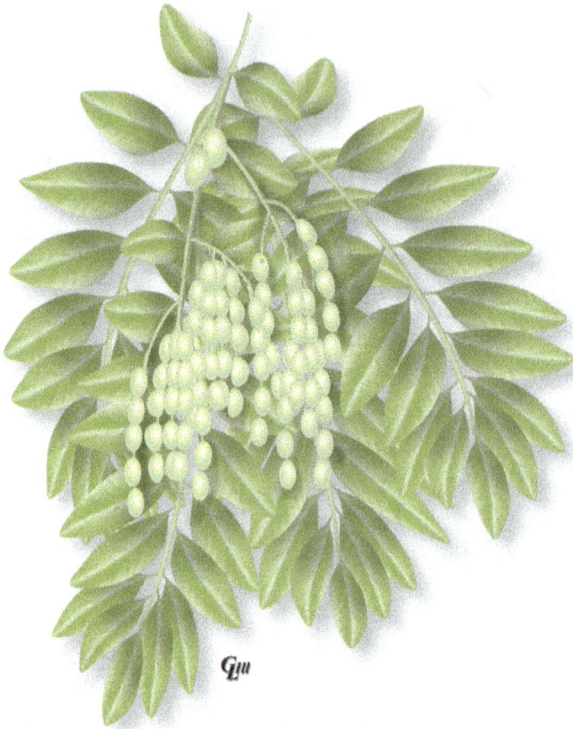

Fig. 21.   Sophora Japonica

5-lipoxygenase inhibitor and COX-1 inhibitor). PS extracts of St. John's Wort (SJW) can be used as a supplementary or even single treatment for depression.

SJW flowers contain its biologically active ingredients hypericin and hyperforin.

SJW may increase CNS serotonin and in very high doses, acts like a monoamine oxidase inhibitor.

Claims: A major constituent, hyperforin, may be used to treat alcoholism (dosage side effects and efficacy are still unclear).

Study findings are variable, but SJW PS supplements may be used by patients with mild to moderate depression.

However, a large study found SJW ineffective in treating major depression.

The suggested dose is 300 mg–600 mg *per os,* once/day of a PS supplements preparation (0.2–0.3 hypericin to 1–4% hyperforin).

SJW may also be useful in treating HIV infection, but there are proven adverse interactions with protease inhibitors and non-nucleoside reverse transcriptase inhibitors (NNRTIs).

A small study indicated that SJW supplements (standardized to hypericin but not to hyperforin) were not effective in relieving symptoms of attention deficit hyperactivity disorder in children.

SJW has shown some possible actions in Parkinson's disease indicating that SJW also has antioxidant active ingredients that may reduce the neuronal degeneration caused by the disease.

Hypericin and pseudohypericin have shown both antiviral and antibacterial activities. These molecules bind non-specifically to viral and cellular membranes and can result in photo-oxidation of the pathogens killing them.

Adverse effects: Minor effects include photosensitivity, dry mouth, constipation, dizziness, confusion and more important side effects may include manic manifestations (in patients with bipolar disorder).

SJW should not be used in pregnant women. Potential adverse interactions may occur with cyclosporine, digoxin, iron supplements, MAOIs, NNRTIs, oral contraceptives, protease inhibitors, SSRIs, tricyclic antidepressants and anticoagulants.

In large doses, SJW is poisonous to cattle, sheep, goats and horses.

Main signs of poisoning are general restlessness and skin irritation. Horses may have symptoms of anorexia and depression (sometimes a comatose state) with dilated pupils (Fig. 22).

Valerian

Valeriana officinalis (Caprifoliaceae) is a perennial flowering plant with heads of sweetly scented pink or white flowers that bloom in the summer months. Valerian flower extracts have been used as a perfume.

Valerian's root and rhizomes (underground stems) contain active ingredients, including valepotriates and pungent, aromatic oils.

Pure extracts of the root are often sold in the form of capsules.

Valerian root has significant sedative and anxiolytic effects. It can also be classified as a drug since its consumption produces a sedative or medicinal effect on the basis of the dosage.

These effects are possibly mediated through the GABA receptor. The amino acid valine is named after the name of the plant.

Known compounds detected in valerian that may contribute to its method of action are

- Flavanones: hesperidin, 6-methylapigenin and linarin,
- Alkaloids: actinidine, chatinine, shyanthine, valerianine, valerine,
- GABA,
- Isovaleric acid,
- Iridoids, including valepotriates: isovaltrate, valtrate,
- Sesquiterpenes (contained in the oil): valerenic acid, hydroxyvalerenic acid and acetoxyvalerenic acid,
- Isovaleramide may be created in the extraction process.

Claims: Valerian is generally used as a week, reliable and safe sedative and as a sleeping aid.

In several studies, valerian improved sleep quality and shortened the time needed to fall asleep.

However, these observations are very difficult to evaluate and quantify; there is insufficient clinical experience (but this is not really a clinical problem) to confirm whether valerian is effective for insomnia.

For mild non-clinical sleeping problems, it could be a mildly effective and a safe solution.

Some people take valerian for headaches, even depression, irregular heartbeat, anxiety or trembling linked to some form of stress.

There is not enough evidence to determine whether valerian may work or give significant advantages for these conditions. Patients may try the PS products and on the basis of their individual response decide whether they want to continue or use a prescription product according to the indication of their physician.

Valerian is usually — as extract or PS supplements — used for short periods of time (four to six weeks); most studies and experiences suggest that it is generally safe.

Adverse effects: Valerian may theoretically prolong the effect of other sedatives (e.g., barbiturates) and — always in theory — affect driving or other activities requiring alertness. It should be used as a single treatment.

It may be more effective in subjects using anti-histamine drugs.

A meta-analysis (how can you make a meta-analysis with different products, administrations and dosages?) published in 2006 in the *American Journal of Medicine* concluded that available evidence indicate that valerian might improve sleep quality without producing side effects.

How you assess sleep quality is a real issue.

Most effects could be individually based.

An article in the *Medical Science Monitor* states indicates that "... based on cellular and animal (again what kind of animal model can you use for getting sleep?) studies as well as human clinical (clinical?) trials there is a role for valerian (including root extract) as useful alternatives in the management of stress and anxiety."

Another systematic review (2007) in the Journal *Sleep Medicine Review*, indicated that valerian is safe but not clinically effective for insomnia.

Actually, valerian is a very good model to discuss some aspects of this field.

Many patented drugs have less evidence than most supplements for efficacy and definitely much lower levels of safety and tolerability.

For Valerian, there is a possible and a very important, individual component that should be considered and respected (see Figure 22).

Zinc

The mineral is required in small quantities in humans and it is essential in multiple metabolic pathways. In many respects, zinc is chemically similar to magnesium: its ion is of similar size and its only common oxidation state is +2.

Dietary sources include oysters, beef and fortified cereals. Zinc is an essential mineral of "exceptional biologic and public health importance". Zinc deficiency affects about two billion people in the developing world and is associated with many diseases.

In children, it causes growth retardation, delayed sexual maturation, infection susceptibility and diarrhea, contributing to the death of about 800,000 children worldwide per year.

Zinc may speed up the healing process after an injury.

It is possibly beneficial to the body's immune system. Zinc deficiency may have effects on all parts of the human immune system.

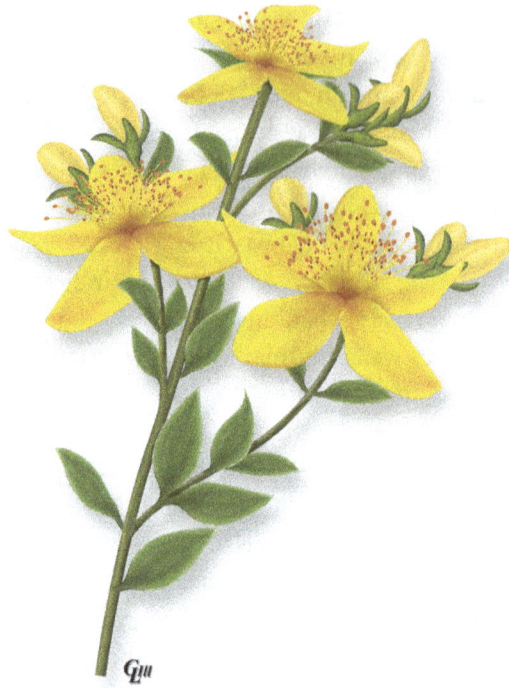

Fig. 22. St. John's Wort

Enzymes with a zinc atom in the reactive center are widespread in biochemistry, such as alcohol dehydrogenase in humans.

Consumption of excess zinc can cause ataxia, lethargy and copper deficiency.

Zinc deficiency has also been associated with a major depressive disorder (MDD), and zinc supplements may be an effective treatment.

Claims: Some experts believe that when taken soon after cold symptoms develop, zinc (used as zinc gluconate or acetate lozenges) may shorten the course of the common cold. Studies are limited — as for any non-patentable product — but zinc even with a limited effect, occurring when it is taken very soon after cold symptoms develop, may reduce the global effect of the common cold.

A one day reduction in individuals' infection of the common cold would considerably reduce the global number with a significant reduction in health costs.

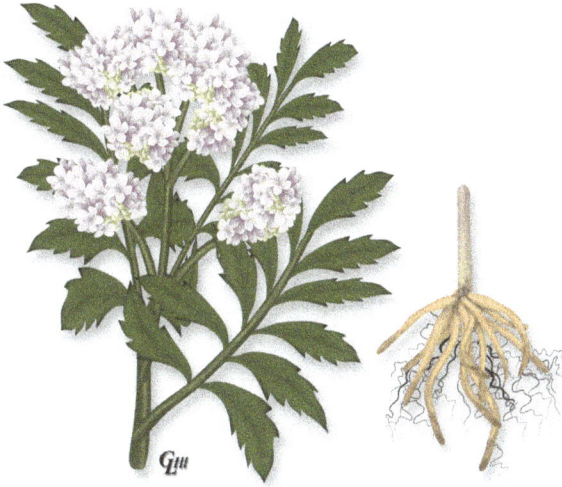

Fig. 23. Valerian

There is stronger evidence that in developing countries, supplements containing zinc 20 mg and iron taken once a week reduce mortality in infants who have diarrhea and respiratory infection.

There is also strong evidence that zinc supplements containing 80 mg and antioxidants once a day slow progression of moderate to severe atrophic (dry form) age-related maculopathy in elderly people.

Adverse effects: Zinc is generally considered safe, but toxicity can develop if high doses are used. Common adverse effects of zinc lozenges include nausea, vomiting, diarrhea, mouth irritation, mouth sores, and bad, metallic taste.

Zinc is a trace metal and can remove other necessary metals from the body; therefore, zinc lozenges should not be taken for more than three weeks.

Some zinc sprays may cause nose and throat irritation.

The effects of certain antibiotics may be altered and decreased by the consumption of zinc supplements.

A study published in 2008 determined that zinc glycinate is the best absorbed of the four dietary supplement types available.

Part 2 — Use of Supplements in Different Clinical Conditions

Cardiovascular Disease

In **cardiovascular disease, Pharma-standard (PS) supplements** can be used in preclinical and preventive applications, borderline problems (hypertension, hyperlipidemia) and clinical conditions.

Safety is essential as these supplements may be used for long periods of time and very often, in concomitance with other products (i.e., antiplatelet agents or anticoagulants, antihypertensives, etc.).

The potential negative interaction with antiplatelet agents is very often very theoretical and practically irrelevant from a clinical point of view.

The interaction with anticoagulants is potentially more serious and significant with potentially severe clinical problems both associated with decreased clotting and increased hemorrhage or bleeding tendency or an increase in clotting that may lead to thrombosis.

Any supplement that could be used by patients or physicians for any cardiovascular conditions (or in any patient with cardiovascular problems requiring medical treatment) should be safe (it should be tested) for its potential thrombogenicity or for its bleeding or anticoagulant facilitating activity.

There are several claims about products that may help decreasing **total lipids,** but only green tea and possibly fish oil products may help (according to several studies) in a significant way.

CP and garlic supplements decrease **triglyceride** levels (in some patients but not without a diet).

High-density lipoprotein (HDL) increase has been shown in studies with garlic and ginseng supplements.

Heart failure has been improved with CoQ10 supplementation. CoQ10 also appears to be useful to fight anthracycline.

CoQ10 is generally decreased in a number of patients using statins and some cholesterol lowering drugs. The decrease in CoQ10 in tissues (including myocardium) is associated with muscular pain and fatigue, and possible heart failure.

Restoring normal CoQ10 levels may be essential in decreasing mortality in patients using statins for a long period of time.

BP has been shown to improve with some fish oil PS supplements (and less, minimally, with garlic). Borderline hypertensive patients had significant benefits by being supplemented with Pycnogenol and in a recent specific study on — otherwise healthy — borderline hypertensive subjects with a grape seed PS supplement.

A global (small) reduction in **lipids** has been suggested with green tea (however, the quantity of reduction is difficult to define and it is probably minimal from a clinical point of view).

Definitely, one green tea (Camellia) PS supplement improves BP and metabolic parameters in borderline subjects with metabolic syndrome (including increased blood pressure).

Atherosclerosis constitutes the greatest challenge in contemporary cardiovascular treatment, due to its complexity and how widespread it is.

It is the mother of all other cardiovascular problems. Atherosclerosis control and treatment is essential for any possible management of most cardiovascular patients.

At the moment, there is not a single treatment for atherosclerosis which, being multifactorial and multifaceted is basically characterized by irregular growth of plaques in the arteries, almost always in hemodynamically important points (i.e., bifurcations of the carotid and coronary arteries in low shear stress parts of the arterial segments).

Atherosclerosis is age-related (but most diseases are age-related and it is difficult to manage or treat age).

It is the most diffuse and demanding (costs, complications and lives) complex of problems. There is evidence that in subjects with increased plasmatic oxstress, the genesis, evolution and progression of plaques is faster and therefore, antioxidants are considered useful to stop progression.

In a recent specific study, results indicated that Pycnogenol+CA (in a specific combination 100+100 mg) decrease the growth of atherosclerotic plaques (carotid, aorta and femoral arteries and, very possibly, at coronary level) independently from a reduction in the major risk factors. The combination seems to control the accumulation of collagen and plaque inflammation.

These studies last years and require a large number of patients.

Studies also indicate that lipids enter the arterial wall in the presence of higher oxidative stress and plaques grow faster in the presence of higher oxidative stress. The combination of CA+Pycnogenol appears to reduce the irregular deposition of collagen in atherosclerotic plaques reducing their progression and controlling the passage to symptomatic stages. This happens in concomitance with a control of altered (increased) oxstress.

Additionally, there is a significant number of subjects that may remain asymptomatic (the plaques do not grow to become clinically important) for years.

The use of an associated antiplatelet agents (i.e., aspirin or ticlopidine) is facilitated in its action by Pycnogenol that has an intrinsic antiplatelet action.

Like **Captain Achab's tear** includes the whole universe and more, a small atherosclerotic plaque includes a universe of life conditions, diseases and historical diseased conditions leading to such complexity that it will take considerable time to define and stop.

At the moment, a more regular incorporations of collagen into the plaque, controlling inflammation and oxstress, seems a very good start to stop the progression of atherosclerosis and single plaques and a significant, safe and easy clinical option to offer to many patients.

Microcirculation changes (i.e., in diabetic microangiopathy, in vasospastic disorders) may be obtained with Pycnogenol and Gingko. Results may be clinically important in most individuals.

Curcumin (as Meriva) may stop the progression of diabetic microangiopathy — and possibly of retinopathy — in longer studies.

Microcirculation studies are the key to evaluate most modern PS supplements and their clinical effects.

Endothelial dysfunction may be improved with Pycnogenol and fish oil, but the results are clinically difficult to evaluate and extrapolate to clinical contexts.

One recent study shows that endothelial function can be improved with Pycnogenol in subjects with severe coronary problems. However, endothelial dysfunction is an early observation in the development of atherosclerosis (i.e., in subjects without plaques) and it is more a risk condition than a real disease which may require treatment. Often, the risk conditions causing endothelial dysfunction (i.e., hypertension, hypercholesterolemia) should be clinically addressed in the first place.

The 'treatment' of endothelial dysfunction — which is not a disease — should not be a main target but an accessory evaluation in the evaluation of PS supplements.

The **risk of myocardial infarction** has been reduced in some important studies with fish oil.

Also, recurrence of MI may be reduced using the proper managements and fish oil.

However, there are studies indicating that the oxidation of fish oil supplements in the intestinal transit may be damaging.

Arrhytmia can also be controlled with fish oil in some patients or controlled with valerian.

Reduction of caloric load and lipid absorption, a metabolic more than a cardiovascular target, has been obtained as a logic step to control atherosclerosis (but it is not a 'real' cardiovascular treatment).

Camellia, the green tea PS supplement, controls all lipids in borderline metabolic syndrome.

Effects on peripheral vascular disease (associated with claudication) have been shown with Ginko PS supplements.

Venous Disease

Both signs and symptoms associated with varicose veins and **CVI** are effectively and safely treated even for long periods with Pycnogenol that is the most powerful compound usable in venous disease.

Sophora japonica is present as an essential component in one of the leading products used for venous disease (Venoruton, Novartis) and it is highly effective and safe.

Grape leaf supplements and CA supplements are also used.

Centella is more effective in advanced stages and in healing venous ulcers.

Pycnogenol has also been effectively used to heal venous ulcers (even in topical formulations).

The main action of Pycnogenol is in its great ability to control edema at capillary level in venous hypertensive microangiopathy.

Diabetic and venous microangiopathies are both 'high-perfusion' microangiopathies and are generally associated to edema.

Edema control at capillary level improves nutrition, perfusion and promotes healing with similar mechanisms.

Lymphatic Disease

At the moment, there is no specific treatment for primary lymphedema. Edema, in lymphatic patients, is characterized by a high level of proteins in the interstitial fluid. Primary lymphedema is very rare and no significant company has invested in a problem that is limited. Postsurgical or post radiotherapy lymphedema is a common observation that requires a complex of treatments. The French oak wood PS supplement Robuvit has recently shown an important action in patients with primary lymphedema controlling signs and symptoms. More studies are in progress.

Sophora Japonica (however, there are no specific products) may also be useful.

Supplements, Thrombosis and Re-Thrombosis Prevention, Thrombogenicity

Nattokinase and Pycnogenol in combination are found in an antithrombotic product (Flite Tabs) that has been tested in long flights as an antithrombotic with good results (however, more subjects are needed).

Pycnogenol is being used in open registries in two studies on recurrent deep venous thrombosis and in retinal thrombosis (to prevent another episode) with results that are better than aspirin (< 5% recurrence in five years).

Pycnogenol also appears to decrease the occurrence of **postthrombotic syndrome**, mainly by controlling postthrombotic edema.

Specific studies on the efficacy and potential clinical value of Pycnogenol as an antithrombotic agent are in progress.

Joint, Bones

There are basically two types of problems (they can be combined) in joint and bone problems due to osteoarthrosis (OA). An inflammatory process may be present and active and may be the main cause of arthrosis.

A mainly degenerative process (i.e., due to excessive weight on the knee) may cause comparable or concomitant OA problems.

The aim of treatments with PS supplements is to decrease pain and stiffness making the patients able to walk and operate again.

OA can be effectively treated with black cohosh PS supplements that improve symptoms in most patients.

Chondroitin sulfate (CS) is also effective (but the positive effects may be minimal in some subjects if the supplement is used as a single treatment). The combination with glucosamine makes most combination supplements effective, well tolerated and practical and may allow many of these patients to avoid long periods of use of NSAIDs with all potential consequences in costs and side effects.

PS supplements with green tea, S-Adenosyl-L-Methionine (SAM), curcumin and Pycnogenol have been used to successfully reduce pain and inflammation.

The effects of treatments may be very individual. In more severe phases with strong inflammation and pain, other 'heavier' treatments may be needed but in 'remission' periods, most supplements are safe, effective, well tolerated and cost-effective.

The short-term target could be improving signs and symptoms and, the long-term target, if possible, could be rebuilding some of the damaged cartilage restoring the cartilage to stages closer to its initial functional physiology and morphology.

To improve joint mobility, stiffness and walking distance without pain, PS supplements allows a significant reduction in costly, time consuming 'conventional' management methods (i.e., physiotherapy, rehabilitation and hospital admission).

New PS products including Meriva (curcumin), boswellia and Pycnogenol have been shown to improve the Karnofsky scale (the global functional ability of patients) and the Western Ontario and McMaster Universities Arthritis Index (WOMAC) score (specifically devised to study

OA with its signs and symptoms) even delaying the need for surgery in some patients.

Feverfew supplements have also been used.

The treatments with supplements should be adapted to each single patient and all the factors aggravating the clinical picture (i.e., excessive weight, a sedentary life) should be also aggressively corrected.

Rheumatoid Arthritis and conditions with a very strong inflammatory component have been treated with success with black cohosh PS supplements.

Finally, a recent study shows that Pycnogenol lowers C-reactive protein and oxidative stress in symptomatic patients with OA.

OA management is one of the most important fields of application for supplements and should be well-known by all physicians and practitioners dealing with these patients.

Menopausal Transition: Women's Health

Signs and symptoms could be controlled on a very individual basis using black cohosh supplements, green tea and Pycnogenol or a Pycnogenol association (Lady Prelox).

Menopause is not a disease but may negatively affect many women. Studies with Pycnogenol show very good effects in pre and postmenopausal women and during the 'menopausal transition'.

Other symptoms like vaginal dryness and small infections, particularly in diabetic menopausal women, were positively affected by a specific PS supplement (Lady Prelox) including Pycnogenol, Rosvita, L-Arginine and L-Citrulline.

Menstrual Symptoms are attenuated (on an individual basis) by black cohosh, feverfew and Pycnogenol.

Estrogenic effects can be obtained with ginseng, but there is a limited number of cases studied so far.

Finally, some recurrent vaginal infections could be treated with goldenseal supplements.

The many aspects of the functional and physiological sexual life of women (including the menopausal transition) should be better explored in all their phases and this could become a very significant field of action for many supplements. New supplements (including ferula) are in advanced phases of development.

Most signs and symptoms are basically an expression of physiology and not pathology and may benefit from 'mild-soft' management with supplements, leaving drugs for more severe, debilitating pathological conditions.

Inflammation

Inflammation is a significant component of most pathological processes that require treatment when excessive and out of control. Chamomile and ginger supplements may reduce both local and systemic, mild inflammatory processes without using more significant, dangerous and costly drugs that may cause side effects.

Some 'bark-steroids' may have a profile comparable to corticosteroids on inflammation but with a weaker physiological action and a less dangerous pattern and frequency of side effects (i.e., boswellia, Pycnogenol, curcumin). They should be considered instead of corticosteroid (for instance, in remission phases when the full action of corticosteroids is not needed).

Fever

Fever is one of the most common signs to be always managed with great attention.

Chamomile and craneberry PS supplements may help. It is possible that other supplements could be used, but this field requires research.

GI and Hepatic Diseases

This is another field of great interest for PS supplements with many effective products available.

Stomach cramps may benefit from chamomile. Indigestion signs have been also treated with chamomile, goldenseal supplements and gastritis (even ulcers in the past) have been treated with chamomile and licorice either in its natural forms or as supplements.

Vomit and nausea (including motion sickness and pregnancy) may be controlled by ginger supplements.

Symptoms of diarrhea can be mitigated with goldenseal supplements.

Acute mild-moderate hepatitis associated to drug treatments or alcohol (and marginally even some cases of initial cirrhosis) can be positively affected by MT supplements and Robuvit (as shown in two recent studies) and by SAM.

Both Liverubin (Alchem) and Robuvit were effective in improving enzyme patterns (normalizing bilirubin and improving albumin) in weeks with a very good safety profile, essential in these patients.

In these cases (there is no established drug or treatment for moderate hepatitis of this kind), the physician should not add the damage potentially caused by a treatment to an already established hepatic failure that may precipitate in case of further damage.

Mushroom poisoning — very dangerous and fast in its evolution — could benefit from high-dosage MT supplements.

However, the number of cases is very limited and the patients are never 'standard' cases. There is a very large variability of clinical conditions.

Asthma

Feverfew has been used in asthma and it could be effective on an individual basis (the patient may try the supplement and judge whether it is effective for his/her situation or not). Pycnogenol has also been used in stable, otherwise healthy patients, with good functional results and improvements in signs and symptoms. A study has also indicated that Pycnogenol may have a histamine-controlling effect that needs to be evaluated in larger clinical studies.

Tracheal burning or irritation, sore throat and other symptoms due to involvement of the upper respiratory tract can be relieved by ginger supplements and expectorants including licorice.

A specific product (Phyto-flu, Alchem, including ginseng and pomegranate) may be effective both for treatment and control and for prevention of viral infections. Studies are in progress.

Weight Loss

It is not a real clinical problem by itself and basically, it is not a disease. Chromium Picolinate (CP) has been used to reduce body fat and for the metabolic control of risk factors: it may increase insulin function.

The supplementation does not help diabetics and the effects on body composition may be minimal.

Camellia (a PS green tea supplement) has been effectively used in subjects with borderline metabolic syndrome with good results in limited studies and absolute safety and tolerability. Pycnogenol also helps in borderline, metabolic syndrome and it had been used with significant results in specific subjects with an inflammatory component (i.e., increased C-reactive protein) and/or increased oxidative stress.

Weight loss cannot be gained with drugs.

There are too many components.

Eating less, eating less junk food and exercising more could be the main key to weight loss.

But we need to have a double blind study to show this concept and an endorsement from Cochrane.

Immune Stimulation

This is not a clinical condition or a disease unless we include subjects with immune depression caused by severe problems, i.e., HIV, radio or chemotherapy.

When using supplements, the meaning of 'immune stimulation' is basically related to make a defence system more efficient in case of a viral aggression (i.e., flu or cold).

CoQ10 supplements, echinacea and ginseng have shown the capacity of increasing the resistance to minor viral infections (cold or flu).

The idea that stimulating the immune system may prevent cancer is a an abstract concept, never shown in a clinical setting or study.

Cold and flu are the most frequent diseases and a prevention method could be very important.

PS supplements including echinacea or ginseng or PS supplements with goldenseal have been shown to be effective in reducing the duration (and severity) of cold; zinc has been studied in several clinical experiences and appears to reduce the duration of cold episodes.

Adding Vitamin C seems to have a minimal effect. Vitamin C should probably be used per periods of time before an episode to have an effect.

The number of subjects with flu or cold, the number of tracheal-bronco-pulmonary complications due to severe flu (including hospital admission, particularly in older, higher risk subjects) has been reduced using colostrum.

Colostrum appeared more effective than the antiflu vaccination and it is very safe.

It is clear that very large studies are needed for these types of evaluations.

Products should be always used considering the context, the basic health of the subject to be supplemented and results should be evaluated on an individual basis.

Even by shortening of one single day, a flu or cold episode would enormously decrease medical costs and problems.

Often that extra day with cold or flu (generally, the last day) is the one that causes more complications and increases costs.

Kidney and Urinary Infections

Craneberry has been successfully used and is recommended for common, mild-moderate and recurrent UTI.

The use of craneberry PS supplements is effective both in reducing the colonization by the most common bacteria, but it is also effective to reduce inflammation after the 'real' bacterial infection is completely treated and there are no detectable bacteria in the urines.

Craneberry is particularly effective in recurrent small infection in healthy subjects (and particularly in women). A severe infection on a patient with other clinical problems should be aggressively treated with the appropriate antibiotic.

Also, craneberry can be used for the post catheterization period when a mix of mild inflammation and infection may persist and cause symptoms.

The administration of craneberry should be continued for some 60 days. Craneberry has no side effect but promotes acidity in urines and it may theoretically promote the formation of uric acid kidney stones in some predisposed individuals. Theoretically, it may interact with anticoagulants.

Concerning the kidney, **cyclosporine nephrotoxicity** and possibly other kinds of nephrotoxicity has been attenuated with fish oil supplements and with gingko.

Benign Prostatic Hyperthrophy

It is a very diffuse condition. Saw palmetto (SP) — in different formulation and with different PS supplements — has been shown to be effective and it is used as a significant treatment in subjects with benign prostatic hypertrophy (BPH).

It is competitive with 'standard' treatments, has no side effects (possibly, just minor diarrhea or headache on an individual basis) and could be an important choice for starting a treatment in case of initial symptoms of BPH or when drug are not tolerated or have caused side effects of intolerance.

The complex Echinacea + SP in PS supplements appears to be more effective than SP alone.

Patients may start with an SP PS supplement and evaluate by themselves the efficacy of the treatment (i.e., on urinary symptoms). It is possible that SP may be effective on an individual basis and some subjects may be less or more responsive to the supplements.

Eye

Gyrate atrophy of the choroid and retina are positively affected by creatine administration. This is a very specialized application of creatine and requires specific competence.

Creatine can also be effective in age-related maculopathy. The retinal microcirculation may be affected by ginkgo (improving flow) and Pycnogenol (with a specific activity on edema control and also improving retinal flow). The evolution of diabetic microangiopathy (at retinal level) can be improved in longer periods using curcumin (as Meriva).

A specific combination (Mirtogenol) has been recently developed for the microcirculation of the eye. This supplement is a combination of standardized bilberry extract (from fresh fruit of *Vaccinium myrtillus*, called Mirtoselect) and Pycnogenol.

Improving the microcirculation may also be effective (in selected patients) in reducing ocular pressure.

The optic nerve is damaged by the higher, chronic intraocular pressures. The decrease in the blood flow to the optic nerve makes this nerve susceptible to the damage induced by the high levels of intraocular pressure.

However, more studies are needed in a larger number of subjects.

Neurology

Neurology is a great, interesting and large field but on the whole disappointing for supplements (but the same could be said for most drug treatments).

The blood–brain barrier (BBB) is a highly selective permeability barrier. It separates the circulating blood in capillaries from the brain extracellular fluid (BECF) in the central nervous system (CNS). The BBB is a structure based on capillary endothelial cells connected by tight junctions with an extremely high electrical resistivity.

The BBB allows the selective passage of water, some gases and lipid-soluble molecules (by passive diffusion).

Selective transport of molecules (using energy) is used for glucose, amino acids and elements that are essential for the functions of the neural network.

The BBB selectively prevents the passage of lipophilic, potential neurotoxins (by an active transport mechanism mediated by P-glycoprotein).

Astrocytes are necessary for the BBB. A small number of regions and areas in the brain, including the circumventricular organs (CVOs), do not have a BBB. Morphologically, the BBB is situated around capillaries and includes tight junctions around the capillaries that do not exist in the normal distal circulation. Endothelial cells restrict the diffusion of microscopic objects (e.g., bacteria) and large or hydrophilic molecules into the cerebrospinal fluid (CSF) but allow the diffusion of small hydrophobic molecules (O_2, CO_2, hormones).

Many supplements do not reach the BBB and most do not pass it. Therefore, experiences are limited and disappointing.

There is some evidence of an efficacy of creatine in **Parkinson** disease.

DHEA has been evaluated in mood disorders with some results.

Insomnia and sleep disorders are improved by DHEA, chamomile supplements, by melatonin and valerian but on an individual basis.

In **Alzheimer's disease,** DHEA has been used with contrasting results (but most treatments do not work in this condition).

In subjects with **dementia,** ginkgo supplements may help. The problem is that ginkgo will improve the arterial flow and microcirculation in the brain, but this does not mean that the cerebral and neurological functions are improved. More flow does not mean more or better function.

Migraine has been treated with some success (individual basis) with feverfew supplements.

Problems related to **jet lag** (sleep disorders, attention deficits, desynchronization, decrease in mental performance, etc.) have been improved with melatonin (as melatonin may improve sleep and rest).

Studies with Pycnogenol indicate that most jet lag related problems may be due to a minimal accumulation of fluid in the brain (as it happens for the lower limbs).

The control of edema may be effective in preventing both cerebral and leg edema (fluid accumulation during long flights) restoring normal cerebral function. The effect on edema is more evident in subjects using antihypertensive drugs that are particularly prone to edema.

Jet lag is an important model (it is not a disease) showing that the regulation of water — possibly causing edema — out of the BBB may actually improve cerebral functions.

Depression (a wide definition of conditions) has been positively affected, in some subjects, with SAM and with PS supplements of SJW.

Mild **anxiety** (also including a wide range of clinical and subclinical conditions) may be easily, safely and effectively affected by sedatives as chamomile and valerian.

Wound Healing

Several products can be used for wound healing; echinacea supplements have shown a significant effect. Also, topical Pycnogenol and Centella/TTFCA have been effectively used for ulcers (both venous due to DVI and diabetic ulcers due to microangiopathy). CA supplements also reduce the formation of cheloids (i.e., in children after burns) and irregular cicatrization.

Platelet Aggregation

Several supplements claim some activity on platelet aggregation. Often the effect is not clinically very relevant and it is not dangerous in case of interactions.

Feverfew and SAM may alter platelet functions. Pycnogenol studies indicate an antiplatelet action that may be synergic with other antiplatelet agents (i.e., aspirin) and may be of clinical interest and value.

More studies and new technology will soon give more results of clinical value.

Diabetes

Diabetes *per se* does not seem affected by most supplements, but these products may either improve diabetic control or make (very occasionally) the control of diabetes more difficult or interfere with the many treatments used by diabetics.

Ginseng supplements may have a significant action on diabetes but need to be evaluated in larger studies.

Generally, the field of PS supplements should have more attention and more targeted research — for this diverse and challenging condition which leads to so many complications and preventable deaths.

However, the push of many **big-pharma** companies in this field — often working as a 'cartel' — make almost impossible to overcome barriers to entry into the market by smaller companies with potentially interesting products. Also, diabetics constitute a 'poor' market. Most diabetics, in most NH systems, receive 'free' treatment, and are therefore unused to spending money on PS supplements.

Antimicrobial Activity

Antimicrobial activity of PS supplements (excluding craneberry with its high specificity for UTI) is not really usable for important clinical applications associated with severe infections, i.e., the theoretic antimicrobial activity of garlic or curcumin have a minimal clinical value.

Tinnitus

Tinnitus (when its origin in vascular due to microcirculatory problems) could be affected by gingko supplements and by Pycnogenol. However, gingko may work only on tinnitus with a significant vascular component (improving the vasospasm in the microcirculation) and therefore is effective only on tinnitus of vascular origin.

Pycnogenol is also effective on the microcirculation and may help reduce edema in a region with minimal vein drainage and no lymphatic component.

Therefore, alterations in the microcirculation (i.e., vasospasm, reduced flow) or cochlear edema should be present (and diagnosed) before using the supplements to have some clinical success. Pycnogenol has shown efficacy in patients with tinnitus and Meniere's syndrome and should be used on an individual basis in these subjects.

Andrology

Some andrological indications (decreased libido and erectile dysfunction or ED) could be positively affected by DHEA and by a specific combination supplement (Prelox).

Prelox is PS supplement, combination of two ingredients, L-Arginine and Pycnogenol.

It has been shown in several studies to increase penile blood flow and release vasospasm.

The product is safe and well tolerated and, in a condition like ED (with so many hormonal, psychological and other components) may have a significant role on an individual basis.

Other Uses of PS Supplements

Some concepts like '**more energy**' or well-being are very difficult to fit in a clinical context and often meaningless.

We do not discuss them in this text focusing on clinical applications.

Athletic performance may be improved with CoQ10, creatine, DHEA, ginseng and with Pycnogenol. However, this is outside the realm of clinical problems and out of the fields of interests for this text. Probably, most dubious supplements in this field are also out of the concept of sport.

Specialists in **cocoonology** or 'longevity' may have a different interest in prolonging life for ever (see the paranoid media attention for Resveratrol that basically has no evidence).

Again, age is not a disease *per se* and Gerovital-like supplements have probably passed their time, but they still have a market.

The use of some supplements for **cancers** (excluding some palliative application) appears very difficult and controversial to manage.

While there is (possibly) a correlation between the use of some supplements in the daily diet, in some populations (i.e., curcumin) and the reduced incidence of some cancers (i.e., colon cancer, prostatic cancer), to transfer these information into clinical steps or using a supplement to decrease the frequency of cancers would require a large amount of time, thousands of patients and aggressive speculations.

In some cancer patients, **side effects from radio or chemotherapy** are reduced by Pycnogenol or curcumin administration (Meriva), but this has nothing to do with the primary neoplastic disease and we must be sure that the supplementary treatment does not interfere with the primary antineoplastic management.

Therefore, **cancers, cancer prevention and treatments** are not discussed in this book. The evidence seems to be very weak and often confined to very basic cellular studies far away from clinical contexts.

Testing PS Supplements & Greendrugs: Organization of Supplement Studies 2013, London & Annecy Panel

Background

Clinical trials

Clinical trials are research studies that prospectively assign human participants or groups of humans to one or more health related interventions to evaluate the effects on health outcomes.

In an observational or registry study, without specific interventions, the investigators observe the subjects and measure their outcomes.

The researchers do not actively manage the study.

Supplement studies

Rules and problems:

Steps:

A — Clearly define fields of activity for supplement studies:

PS supplements should be mainly used for preclinical and borderline conditions or risk conditions.

B — Studies should produce comparative data or use comparative backgrounds and historical data for comparable subjects.

C — Supplements should help manage a risk condition or a pre/ subclinical problem. Supplements are not used as drugs for specific claim as treatments.

Standard operating procedures (SOPs)

A — Suggest to patients or subjects at risk, the supplement use (do not prescribe) or supplement options.

The patient or his/her caregiver will decide.

B — Supplements are used on top of 'standard, best management/ care' for that condition.

C — Supplements should not interfere with other treatments.

D — Time periods of follow up may be variable, as a range, not prefixed.

The supplement should be administered as long as needed to see results or changes.

E — Type of evaluation:

(I) Retrospective analysis.

(II) Non-interventional registry.

(III) Observational study without specific interventions.

F — Aim of the studies: evaluate compliance in use of supplements as a resulting critical factor:

Additional information:

- How many subjects are willing to initiate treatment?
- How many subjects will follow treatment as they find benefits?
- How many subjects want to continue supplementation?

Note: For these studies, there should be

- No defined group allocation,
- No randomization,
- No placebo as these conditions necessarily lead to good clinical practice (GCP) studies.

Open label. Patients always know what the supplementation, treatment, management is and what it can do.

The net effect is the supplement action plus a possible placebo action.

Comment: the placebo effect is usually overconsidered and overevaluated in most studies.

It should be positively managed in this type of evaluation.

This conduct for supplement studies also resembles much better an actual preclinical or clinical use with all its implications.

Most of the GCP studies are actually very artificial with defined age and sex definitions and other characteristics that are rarely comparable with real, broad clinical use.

Data are analyzed after a period of study when sufficient evidence is available or when is possible or if limited by funds.

Characteristics of the study:

Supplement studies should be generally:

- Small scale,
- Independent,
- One-center studies,
- Product (supplement) is not directly supplied,
- Products are generally available in the market,
- Patients get or buy the supplement product.

The limited costs should allow anybody in the medical field to plan and organize these studies.

Some studies could be organized by patients or consumers or researchers that have an interest in the problem.

These studies could be very useful particularly in countries with limited budgets and when doctors and group of doctors have limited funds and resources; they may be able to use the (locally produced) supplements instead of importing more expensive products.

Good Clinical practice (GCP) (due to costs and complexity) can only be organized by companies or important institutions with huge costs.

Costly studies are only organized in view of high revenues.

Presence of external study reviewers.

The definition of the role and activity of a possible, international '*super partes*' committee is in progress.

Sponsors/cro (contract research organization) usually is not available and generally is not used to reduce costs.

Conflict of interest: no conflict is a major point.

Advantages of 'supplement' studies:

- Speed,
- Low cost,
- Available for small centers, single physicians, low-budget institutions,
- Local studies may evaluate local, natural products.

Exclusion: In case of clinical problems and clinically significant conditions, it is important to consider **GCP** studies.

When a supplement is intended to treat specific clinical conditions and a study is planned to have a claim, GCP studies should be planned.

Basically, in this situation, the product is not a supplement anymore.

When looking for definite **claims**, GCP studies are needed particularly when it is not possible to organize pilot, open-label studies.

Informed consent (IC) is now needed before any medical action, investigation, procedure or protocol.

It is not specific for this kind of evaluation.

For a supplement registry, you should not ask for another one, particularly if the patient decides to use the supplement by himself.

PS-Supplements; Points to Evaluate

The 150 Factor: Most PS supplements in their historical formats have been tested and evaluated with a factor of 150/1 (subjects or patients) in comparison with 'normal', patented, prescription drugs and are therefore, by definition, safer.

Supplements do not need prescriptions because they are considered safe and easy to use. This is not always the case but it is an important assumption to be validated and verified for each supplement and each application.

The one-shot, one application factor for patented-industrial, prescription drugs makes them more 'specialized' for single applications, and for selected groups of patients.

Therefore, these products tend to be limited in experience and may be a source of problems if applied in a setting that is not exactly corresponding to its specific, defined application (as seen in a clinical trial).

Animal studies and cell models. Animal studies are basically useless unless required to assess safety (even for safety, these models are questionable).

Efficacy cannot be assessed with animal models or cells and the experience cannot be transferred to humans.

Diet, intestinal processing, and absorption and metabolism of most complex supplements are completely different in different species.

It is better not to mention animal models to confuse customers (i.e., cancer cells grow slower with some supplements).

More than useless, these statements can be demeaning or dangerous and cause confusion. They may even determine or facilitate avoidance of 'proven' standard treatments.

Complex versus single molecules. Supplements are usually complex blends of molecules more that a single molecule (as most 'patented', prescription drugs).

It is their weakness and their strength.

It is possible that within a complex supplement, some molecules have a direct clinical effect and others facilitate either absorption, metabolism or the clinical effects or they may protect healthy organs and cells from damage.

Terminology

In dealing with supplements, particularly PS supplements, there are some demeaning words to avoid now when writing or speaking.

It is important to limit confusion and avoid degrading the products.

Phytotherapy is something else, nothing to do with pharmaceutical formulations or PS supplements.

It may include the TRADITIONAL use of unprocessed plants without well-defined standards in dosages or preparations.

'**Alternative**' is really misleading and gives most people and physicians bad feelings. There is nothing alternative in most PS supplements or in their applications. It is simply medicine and pharmaceutical science at its best.

'**Natural**' is also to avoid. Natural has nothing to do with PS supplements that have been produced with a complex and often costly process including standardization. The original natural product may be far away and completely different.

'**Traditional**' also sounds really bad.

Popular is also to be avoided. It does not mean anything. Most of the PS supplements now available have important historical (more than traditional) roots but minimal traditional ties and are derived from a contemporary, complex, costly and long pharmaceutical and industrial evolution.

'**Well-being**' — **really abused** — does not mean anything from a physiological or clinical point of view.

Any claim of 'inducing well-being' should be dismissed with decision and seen with suspicion.

Well-being, if there is anything with this name in medicine, is also very personal.

It cannot be reached with supplements or drugs. At least it should not. After using some drugs, some people may improve their feeling of well-being, but from a medical point of view that may be in a more dangerous situation of bad being.

The mention of well-being is often associated with shamanic intentions from a scientific or clinical perspective.

'**Longevity**' also is a confusing, misleading and abused concept. You cannot increase individual longevity as nobody knows the number of years you may have to live.

It can only be a generic concept related to the average lifespan within a population.

Making telomeres longer in worms or rats does not add very much to our life.

There is **not a single drug or supplement** that can claim to change longevity.

In **summary, language and culture changes** should be significant tools to develop a new system to promote and market PS supplements.

They should be more linked to physiology and to the medical field with all its aspects and basic rules including the important pharmaceutical processes that produce them.

Supplements, by definition, are intrinsically safe, they do not need prescriptions. It is almost impossible to kill yourself with a PS supplements or be killed, by mistake, by supplements. Phytotherapy, on the contrary, may kill.

In USA only, some 15 subjects/year are actually killed by more dangerous phytoproducts (i.e., ephedra, a medicinal preparation from the plant Ephedra sinica) used for weight loss. Concerns regarding the safety of ephedra supplements led the FDA to ban the sale of ephedra-containing supplements in the United States in 2004.

This ban was challenged by supplement manufacturers but eventually maintained.

A review of ephedra-related adverse reactions, published in the New England Journal of Medicine in 2000, found a number of cases of sudden cardiac death or severe disability resulting from ephedra use, many of which occurred in young adults using ephedra in the labeled dosages.

Therefore, all PS supplements should be safe and should not put the patient in any acute risk.

Supplements are often **effective on an individual basis** (this is very important in the age of individualized medicine) and they are a defined individual choice (supplements are not usually provided by healthcare systems), to buy personally, at significant costs.

A choice that costs is always an important choice to respect.

PS supplements should have (with the same product) the same consistent effects, time after time. Patients have the full opportunity to evaluate by themselves the possible positive effects and to decide whether using supplements will be beneficial to their health.

Who is your customer?

Communication to physicians and pharmacists is the key form of promotion for many supplement producers.

However, **the real customer for supplements is the user, the patient.**

Physicians and pharmacists are just facilitators.

The most important level of attention for supplement producers is towards their actual customers who buy the product expecting an effect and who deserve complete attention and frankness.

General Precautions

The US Food and Drug Administration (FDA) recommends consumers to inform their healthcare providers about supplements they are taking as some supplements may not be completely risk-free under certain circumstances (i.e., when patients are also using other products) or may interact with prescription and over-the-counter medicines.

In conclusion, ideally, a PS supplement should not cause problems even with accidental overdoses and should be declared safe and usable without prescription.

Combination products have a significant possibility of application at the moment and more so in the near future.

Many PS supplements now include more that one product. The trend and market are increasing.

The safety of each single product should not be compromised by the combined use with another safe product. But safety, tolerability and potential interaction studies as the first step are still needed for each new combination, even before efficacy studies.

New Evaluations in Progress

Most supplements are a **combination of several compounds**. The cocktails are mostly effective when they include the full combination of compounds. The use of solvents or other complex pharmaceutical methods to extract single, separate elements from the combinations may produce a non-natural compound that is not on the list of supplements (as it may include remnants of solvent or other extracting fractions).

The product could be significantly different from the original complex and expose patients to potentially unknown effects.

The **metabolic pool** is a developing concept including all aspects involving the interactions between the PS supplement and the metabolic pathways.

The metabolic pool and pathways could be completely different among different animals — particularly for complex cocktails of products/ substances — and make animal studies mostly irrelevant.

The interactions in the pool may happen at intestinal level (i.e., altering absorption, competing for absorption of significant nutritional or toxic elements), with a direct interaction with organs in the venous bloodstream before a first pass effect, with an interaction of the complex or single elements after a first pass effect with partial or complete metabolization of some of the components (altering the composition of the complex). Also, protein or cellular binding and transport, extraction of significant elements from the bloodstream and organs could happen. The metabolic pool model must finally consider the late, possible actions of some remnants either metabolized or unmetabolized and the possible accumulation in specific storage elements (i.e., fat).

The model of the single pharma molecule, generally acting on specific receptors (as proposed for most prescription drugs), with a defined, constant metabolism in standard conditions is not valid for most supplements due to their pharmacological complexity.

The model of the single molecule, selective drug is generally associated to a greater specificity — and very selective activity — and to a greater danger of significant side effects.

The therapeutic range between collateral damage and pharmacological effect is a significant characteristic of molecular drugs, not shared by supplement complexes (lower efficacy, less specific, minimal danger of side effects).

For each supplement, a specific metabolic pool should be defined and evaluated in the next few years.

Evaluation of Thrombogenicity and Compatibility with Anticoagulants or Antiplatlet Agents

Anticoagulants are used very often in a larger number of subjects (with three main indications: thrombosis/embolism, valvular or device anticoagulation, fibrillation and cardiac prevention).

The number of subjects using oral anticoagulants is increasing as is, the number of subjects undergoing heparin prophylaxis (low molecular

weight heparins and new heparins/heparinoids) is increasing. It is impera-
tive, in the next few years, to define the **antithrombogenetic** or **prothrom-
bogenic** activity of most supplements with specific tests.

Also, the number of subjects > 50 using antiplatelet agents is becoming astronomical and possible interactions with antiplatelet agents should
be evaluated.

Preventing **bleeding** (at every level, i.e., at retinal level in diabetics or
in the brain) or unwanted **clotting** (i.e., causing stroke of myocardial
infarction) may reduce a significant number of events and medical, personal and social costs.

Therefore the safety evaluation protocols for PS supplements should
now include the thrombogenesis aspect as it is likely that a great number
of subjects using anticoagulants may use supplements, often, even without
medical prescription or suggestions.

Interactions with other commonly used drugs (antihypertensive,
cholesterol-lowering drugs, anti-diabetic agents) should be evaluated.

The general, individual safety, and the absolute safety of supplements
is broadly valid for subjects not using other drugs/products and without
associated clinical conditions but cannot be defined or granted for patients
using a mix of drugs, i.e., subjects with kidney or liver impairment may
have a different response to some PS supplements that should be considered by a clinician.

Many of our patients (>35% for age >55), even in absence of significant symptoms have to use, on the basis of prescriptions, an antiplatelet
agent, an antihypertensive drug and a lipid-lowering agent.

Therefore, a healthy subject may buy a supplement and use it without
problems of safety, but patients should always talk with their clinician and
ask whether the use of the supplement is appropriate.

The Safety 150/Factor: Safety Table

Tolerability and safety should be the first concern for any PS supplement.
Any study should include as a preliminary step the safety evaluation.
Table 1 (including the seven pillars of safety) can be used as a reference
(Belcaro, 2014).

Table 1:   The tolerability/safety scale: The seven pillars of tolerability.

Safety factor Items	Scale Score Range	0	1	2	3
1. Tolerability	0–3	Very good	Minimal	Significant	Severe
2. Doses assumed	0–3	100%	95–99%	75–94	<75%
3. Side effects	0–3	None	Minimal	Significant	Severe
4. Suspension of treatment	0–3	No	1 dose	>5 doses	Block
5. Treatment subjectively unpleasant	0–3	No	Minimal	Significant	Severe
6. Need for medical attention	0–3	No	Minimal (discussion)	Prescription treatment	Hospital admission
7. Would continue supplementation?	0–3	Yes	If advised	Only if needed	No

The **traditional (better, historical)** use of most products for ages is a significant and clinically important historical evaluation. In centuries of use, any possible side effect or intolerance not only has been noted and has emerged but also has been observed and confirmed several times.

Most — if not all side effects — have been observed and reported and are generally incorporated into the historical profile of the product or extract in its different forms even when the product has not been used as a real PS supplement.

The different side effects and tolerability stories of different extracts and formats are also generally known.

Not a single 'patented' drug, usually used for a specific, single defined use or for a limited range of clinical applications could have the safety profile of any of these **historical** products.

Generally, the **safety/tolerability** profile of any of the historical popular supplements, even not in a PS format, could be at least **some 150 times more validated**, stronger and wider that any 'modern' patented drug.

These 'patented' drugs, tested in a relatively small number of subjects (for short periods of time), in very standard conditions have not been exposed to all the possible human, clinical genetic, interactive combinations and backgrounds that may originate safety or tolerability problems.

Most of the historical products, when found effective in managing one problem, have also been empirically used for similar clinical problems and conditions expanding the experience of these historical products and their safety/tolerability profile.

Not a single 'patented,' designer drug has been tested for so long and so widely and for so many conditions and therefore, not a single 'modern' drug could and will never have this sort of safety/tolerability profile.

Modern drugs last as long as their patent and are in the market at the most for a few decades without any possibility of acquiring this sort of profile. They may be dismissed before they can cause a rare complication.

The only possible exception is aspirin or acetylsalicylic acid (ASA) that has a very wide range of applications and a long standing, historical and popular background.

Of course, these clinical, simple evaluative steps (the seven pillars) should be always associated to a **complete laboratory evaluation** according to need and to specific target organs for each supplement.

If the total is <1, the tolerability/safety is considered optimal.

If the total is >5 and <10, the tolerability/safety is not good and requires a specific safety study.

In case of score >7, supplementation should be questioned and standards, dosages and need for supplementation should be reconsidered and suspended until full documentation is available.

Conclusions

The **supplement world** needs a change and a defined organization with new rules.

At the moment, this field is a mix of good and bad products, and good and bad informations.

Specific research should define clinical aspects for each supplement.

The clinical view is the key. Supplements can only be effectively used by professionals with a strong clinical background.

The evidence for supplement activity should have specific rules. Most of the clinical journals, at the moment, claiming evidence for industrial 'patented' drugs are heavily sponsored by the drug industry.

Pharmaceutical companies will spend millions on patented products that will offer even a minimal benefit, possibly very marginal and not too different from valerian or other extracts or supplements that cannot be protected by a patent.

The supplement world is often therefore excluded or badly tolerated.

The evolution of PS supplements may also consider the production of low-cost (non-patented) products in low-income countries to be used, when and if possible, as possible alternatives to 'patented', more expensive, imported drugs.

In medicine, evidence is only found when and if there is a very high commercial advantage. The industry of PS supplements generally defines a limited, small, relatively low-profit market — with limited patenting possibility — and cannot produce expensive research and therefore strong evidence.

Presentation of Prof. Umberto Cornelli

The purpose of this volume is a rapid analysis of PS products of common use as food supplements. These compounds, although very different in terms of composition, are in all respects *Physiological modulators* (PH; J.A. Olson, J Nutr, 1996) since they are natural derivatives, not produced by chemical synthesis (Physiological) and can adjust some functions of our body (Modulators). Their activity can be beneficial and theoretically, rarely, also toxic depending upon the intrinsic characteristics and dosage. Unfortunately, the official texts of Pharmacology devote to these products only a few lines, often limited to vitamins and minerals. Many of these products have been used for millennia (e.g., extracts of *Ginkgo biloba or Serenoa repens, Centella asiatica*), whereas some others (e.g., CoQ10, *Silybum marianum*) came in into use during the last century.

One important aspect has to be considered in relation to the plant derivatives: they are produced by the given organism for self protection against invading microorganisms and predators (e.g., fungi, bacteria, insects, etc.) and are potentially toxic for the invaders; minerals and trace minerals are part of the biological environment and taken from the soil for enzymatic and non-enzymatic reactions necessary for the growth and survival of every organism.

All the PS supplements derived from the vegetal world have been subjected to chemical analysis to standardize their contents in the attempt to isolate the active principles and those that are known to be toxic. These investigations are very complex and have revealed the presence of differences due to the characteristics of the various species, as well as the methods of cultivation and harvest times.

From these characteristics emerge the fact that standardization of PS can be carried out only by specialized producers equipped with chemical/physical/pharmacological methods following the essential prerequisite of GMP.

The first part of the book describes the general characteristics of PS (composition, biological and clinical activity), while the second part outlines the clinical uses in different diseases, underlining those aimed to the "proof of concept".

A chapter is devoted to focusing on some of the key elements for a correct study and nomenclature of these products. The book may orient health professionals (doctors, pharmacists, nutritionists, dieticians) in this universe that is constantly changing and unfortunately prone to easy sophistication. The International Regulatory Agencies have for decades been controlling the production processes and claims which must be very selective and specific.

Conclusions

Undoubtedly, the use of physiological modulators (PM) — generally corresponding to most PS supplements — may improve health, a right for every subject.

However, very often these compounds are sold with the pretended aim of solving pathological problems, clinical and risk conditions (e.g., senile dementia, ALS) that cannot be cured by valid 'common' or standard therapies. In the majority of the controlled trials in these pathologies, the activity was limited.

In many other diseases (e.g., BPH, diabetes, venous disease), the use of PS clearly reduces or prevents symptoms in the same way or even better than synthetic drugs.

In general, since they are able to modify biological functions, they must be used properly within a defined clinical context.

This caution implies knowledge of their properties, particularly by physicians and some 'health care experts' who are often in contact with patients without having the necessary knowledge to suggest or prohibit their intake. Often the consumer increases dosages to achieve an effect, or to associate more compounds in the mistaken belief that the PS are free of toxicity.

This book may help health professionals to decide on the best opportunities to use or not use PS supplements.

From our analysis of the literature and clinical experience, the following four basic concepts should be considered:

- The products have to come from certified producers that ensure product standardization in terms of GMP.
- The interactions with the basic therapy, in particular, in patients with diabetes, hypertension, and those treated with anticoagulants or CNS drugs. In these cases, limited dosages of PS supplements should be used.

- The third point is related to the associations of various PS. The combination of different products may end up with a synergistic effect both for activity and toxicity. Therefore, before using two formulations (e.g., fish oil, *Camellia sinensis*), one must be certain about the clinical activity of the compounds. When formulas are a mixture of many PS, the best is to avoid their use and shift to a single PS.
- It is important to use PS with demonstrated clinical activity as meta-analysis studies — if available — refer to compounds produced in a different way and not sufficiently comparable. On the other hand, it is easy to understand that the traditional use of many of these derivatives is based on products that are very different from those used by our ancestors since they were using antique and obsolete production methods

Why to use them? The answer is ... why not?

And the solution can come from the clinical evidence only. Many times PS improves the conditions of the patients and achieve results that cannot be obtained with drugs. Time and research will produce appropriate reasons for these improvements, but we must be free from preconceptions.

Index

www.ingramcontent.com/pod-product-compliance
Lightning Source LLC
Chambersburg PA
CBHW052013270326
41929CB00015B/2894